Trauma Texts

These chapters, gathered from two special issues of the journal *Life Writing*, take up a major theme of recent work in the Humanities: Trauma. Autobiography has had a major role to play in this 'age of trauma', and these essays turn to diverse contexts that have received little attention to date: partition narratives in India, Cambodian and Iranian rap, refugee letters from Nauru, graffiti in Tanzania, and the silent spaces of trauma in Chile and Guantanamo. The contexts and media of these autobiographical trauma texts are diverse, yet they are linked by attention to questions of who gets to speak/write/inscribe autobiographically and how and where and why, and how can silences in the wake of traumatic experiences be read. These essays deliberately set out to establish some new fields for research in trauma studies by reaching out to a broader global context, into various texts, media and artifacts, representing diverse histories with specific attention to different voices, bodies, memories and subjectivities. This collection addresses the contemporary circuits of trauma story, and the media and icons and narratives that carry trauma story to political effect and emotional affect.

This book was previously published as two special issues of *Life Writing*.

Gillian Whitlock is Professor in English Media Studies and Art History at the University of Queensland. He specialises in comparative and postcolonial approaches to life writing.

Kate Douglas is Senior Lecturer in English, Creative Writing and Australian Studies at the Flinders University of South Australia who specialises in life writing, trauma and memory theory.

Trauma Texts

Edited by Gillian Whitlock and Kate Douglas

Routledge
Taylor & Francis Group
LONDON AND NEW YORK

First published 2009 by Routledge
2 Park Square, Milton Park, Abingdon, Oxfordshire OX14 4RN

Simultaneously published in the USA and Canada
by Routledge
711 Third Avenue, New York, NY 10017

Routledge is an imprint of the Taylor & Francis Group, an informa business

Typeset in Times by Value Chain, India

British Library Cataloguing in Publication Data
A catalogue record for this book is available from the British Library

ISBN 978-0-415-48300-1 (hbk)
ISBN 978-0-415-85317-0 (pbk)

Contents

1 Introduction: Trauma Texts: Reading Trauma in the Twenty-First Century 1
Kate Douglas and Gillian Whitlock

2 A Transnational Hip Hop Nation: praCh, Cambodia, and Memorialising the Killing Fields 9
Cathy Schlund-Vials

3 Karibu Mwanza: Drawings by Tanzanian Street Children 26
Marcus Wiencke

4 Testimonio and Telling: Women's Narratives of Genocide, Torture and Political Imprisonment in Post-Suharto Indonesia 43
Annie Pohlman

5 Fifty Years On: Melancholic (Re)collections and Women's Voices from the Partition of India 57
Terri Tomsky

6 I Must Know: Re-membering Native Women in the CAVNET_IW Community 75
Jane Haladay

7 Putting Site Back into Trauma Studies: A Study of Five Detention and Torture Centres in Santiago, Chile 91
Peter Read and Marivic Wyndham

8 Textual Traumata: Letters to Lindy Chamberlain 109
Deborah Staines

9 Vulnerable Children, Disposable Mothers: Holocaust and Stolen Generations Memoirs of Childhood 127
Rosanne Kennedy

10 Letters from Nauru 151
Gillian Whitlock

11 Hostile Witness: Torture Testimony in the War on Terror 166
Nina Philadelphoff-Puren

12 From Grief to Grievance: Ethics and Politics in the Testimony of Anti-War Mothers 184
Cynthia G. Franklin and Laura E. Lyons

Index 198

Introduction: Reading Trauma in the Twenty-First Century

Kate Douglas and Gillian Whitlock

In her genealogical approach to the study of trauma, Ruth Leys situates the most recent turn to trauma studies across a range of disciplines and in relation to the waxing and waning of interest in trauma over the course of more than a century. Leys is a useful place to begin, for she reminds us that the current surge in trauma studies is distinctively shaped by politics, culture and history in and of the present, and embedded within an intellectual history that goes back to the origins of psychoanalysis in European modernity. What we have seen in these past two decades, then, draws deeply on debates and therapies that have emerged variously: in the rise of psychoanalysis in the years after 1900; the phenomenon of 'shell shock' after World War I; the recognition of post-traumatic stress disorder amongst veterans in the wake of the Vietnam War, and feminist campaigns in the 1970s concerning sexual abuse in children. Although the germinal texts in theorising trauma and representation in the recent past have focused on the Holocaust – for example Dominick LaCapra, Shosanna Felman and Dori Laub, and Cathy Caruth – and the long-term effects of trauma on survivors of the Nazi genocide was evident in the aftermath of World War II, the Holocaust did not trigger the recent upsurge of trauma studies. Ironically, the history of trauma itself is marked by an alternation between episodes of forgetting and remembering, as the experiences of one generation of psychiatrists have been neglected only to be revived at a later time: 'just as it took World War II to "remember" the lessons of World War I, so it took the experience of Vietnam to "remember" the lessons of World War II, including the psychiatric lessons of the Holocaust' (Leys, 15).

A vigorous and widespread turn to the practice and theory of life writing (a term that covers biography, autobiography and variants and mutations of both) has occurred along with this most recent emergence of trauma studies. The Greek root of trauma is 'wound', and the experience of trauma is an overwhelming and self-shattering event that is frequently theorised as unspeakable, resistant to representation. Trauma, suggests Leigh Gilmore, takes autobiography to the limits of representation. Yet life writing thrives here at the limits, and Gilmore's book considers the aesthetic forms and cultural practices of traumatic life narrative as a distinctively *fin de siècle* phenomenon. She identifies a series of forces at play in and around this convergence of the memoir boom and trauma studies: social and political movements since the 1960s around issues of race, sexuality, class, gender and ethnicity have authorised new subjects and identifications for autobiography, and licensed the telling of previously hidden stories. The culture of confession in the mass media further elicits personal narratives of trauma, suffering and recovery. There is now a market for personal story and a proliferation and innovation in genres of creative non-fiction that expand those with stories to tell, and those with the desire to read life writing.

We see expressed in the studies of trauma narrative and critique that emerged early this century by Gilmore, Nancy K. Miller and Jason Tougaw, Kelly Oliver, and Ruth Leys a series of reservations about the uses of autobiography in this 'age of trauma': 'trauma' has become a 'portmanteau' term that covers a variety of disparate experiences; the 'addiction' to narratives of pain and suffering, and the vogue of violent emotion and shocking events; and the migration of private zones of the body into public domains,

> [I]n a culture of trauma, accounts of extreme situations sell books. Narratives of illness, sexual abuse, torture or the death of loved ones have come to rival the classic, heroic adventure as a test of limits that offers the reader the suspicious thrill of borrowed emotion. (Miller and Tougaw, 2)

Scholarly work on testimony, memoir, witnessing and empathy has critically examined the dynamics of production and consumption of the genres that are carriers of trauma story (for example, Kay Schaffer and Sidonie Smith, Patricia Yaeger, and Gillian Whitlock) and critics have become increasingly concerned about the uses and abuses of empathic engagement with life story. Oliver asks when does a trauma story promote 'pornographic seeing' which makes the other into an object or spectacle, there for the viewer's/reader's pleasure, possessed by the subject's gaze? (156) For Yaeger these questions are especially acute when we consider the burgeoning field of academic writing about trauma:

> We inhabit an academic world that is busy consuming trauma – eating, swallowing, perusing, consuming, exchanging, circulating, creating professional connections – through stories about the dead . . . [w]hat happens when we 'textualize' bodies, when we write about other people's deaths (or other people's cultures) as something one 'reads'? (29)

All of these questions remain sharp and relevant in discussions about life narrative and trauma now. Studies that emerged early this century have about them the air of a retrospective account; a perspective that characterised trauma as a *fin de siècle* preoccupation that was, perhaps, on the edge of running its course and becoming '*fin*'. What happened was an 'event' that has, if anything, accelerated and redefined trauma narrative: '"event" is the "dominant term in trauma discourse, perhaps the most frequently deployed and most ambiguous term of all, universally chosen to refer to what really happens'(Miller and Tougaw, 19). At the end of the introduction to Miller and Tougaw's *Extremities* we find this record of the event that irrevocably reshaped their subject: 'We complete the editing of this manuscript in the aftermath of the World Trade Center's destruction: September 11, 2001. This tragic overture to the twenty-first century has changed the context of this book, jarred our perspective. We are only beginning to take the measure of the new testimonies to loss, the new contexts of traumatic experience that this event has produced' (20). The events of 9/11 made what was (arguably) a swan song of the century just past into an overture for the new. In the context of trauma studies at least, a new 'jarred' perspective and a sense of precarious life emerges. Several things are clear: the dynamics of self-fashioning and the textual cultures of life narrative changed in the course of the 'war on terror', and autobiographers have been called upon to transform the book, the page and the word to make radical uses of the verbal and visual forms and spaces of life narrative (Whitlock, 201). The events of 9/11 authorise new subjects of trauma narrative and so, for example, E. Ann Kaplan begins her study of the cultural politics of trauma personally, with her own experience of post-traumatic stress as a New Yorker whose neighbourhood includes Soho, and as a child in England during World War II. A proliferation of traumatic story and academic writing about it takes a distinctive turn in this new century in the wake of the catastrophic 'wounding' of New York.

This is the context for *Trauma Texts*. We set out to explore academic work on trauma and life narrative now, with a view to seeding debate as well as surveying the field. Those concerns about the ethics of testimony and witnessing, the commodification of traumatic story, and politics of recognition that shape this field of research and writing remain. We have, however, set out to bring some new contexts into view, moving beyond the neighbourhoods of New York and Euro-American contexts more generally. This takes up some challenges triggered by Jill Bennett and Rosanne Kennedy in their edition *World Memory*, which recognises the contribution of psychoanalysis and the Holocaust to developing the framework for trauma studies and at the same time calls for a transformation of the field to embrace a changing global context: trauma studies in the humanities 'must move beyond its focus on Euro-American events and experiences, towards a study of memory that takes as its starting point the multicultural and diasporic nature of contemporary culture' (5). Bennett and Kennedy argue that the events of 9/11 further underline the need to develop critical analysis of differential and intercultural relations and situate the study of trauma in more global political frameworks. As essays in this collection suggest (for example, Kennedy, Read and Wyndham, and Pohlman), insights and the language of trauma studies generated by Holocaust studies are not superseded here but rather relocated, and integrated into comparative perspectives that travel south and into various cultural frameworks and traditions. In *Trauma Texts* we have deliberately set out to travel: to carry thinking about life narrative and trauma across generations, into various texts, media and artifacts, representing diverse histories within nation and beyond, and with specific attention to voices, bodies, memories, sites and subjectivities. Our purpose is to establish dialogues between some of the existing and traditional locations, subjects and methodologies of trauma scholarship, and other contexts, histories and memories that have remained relatively obscure despite the recent surge of scholarly work.

In 'A Transnational Hip Hop Nation: praCh, Cambodia and Memorialising the Killing Fields', Cathy Schlund-Vials examines the memorialising in youth culture of 'the Killing Fields', a genocide engineered by Pol Pot and the Khmer Rouge regime in Cambodia between 1975 and 1979. The Cambodian American rapper and refugee praCh makes hip-hop CDs in his parents' garage in California; his lyrics are in English and Khmer, and based on stories told to him by his family members and Khmer Rouge propaganda speeches. Bootlegged versions of this hip-hop memoir were played on Phnom Penh radio and he became a number-one music artist. Although praCh had not been in Cambodia since he was a toddler, his commemoration of the Killing Fields resonated with Khmer youth. praCh's lyrics and rhythms are a distinctive transnational and generational testimony which negotiate multiple forms of traumatic memory through remembrance and reconciliation, and reclaim Khmer artistic forms (such as pin peat) that were destroyed during the Khmer Rouge regime. Schlund-Vials suggests that contemporary autobiographical discourses of trauma are more syncretic than they may at first appear, and that transnational and diasporic youth cultures have a distinctive role to play in their hybrid new forms, audiences and embodiments. This concern with trauma narrative in youth cultures is taken up very differently in Markus Wiencke's chapter. Wiencke introduces new graphic texts to trauma study: street kids' graphics from Tanzania. This essay draws on different disciplinary perspectives (psychology and social anthropology) and scholarly traditions (German scholarship on the concept of 'life world') to approach these drawings in ways that respect the subjective experience of the street children themselves. Together these two chapters introduce some new media, contexts and methodologies in seeing, hearing and reading trauma narrative in youth cultures.

The following chapters take up issues related to voice, trauma and gender. In 'Testimonio and Telling Women's Narratives of Genocide, Torture and Political Imprisonment in Post-Suharto Indonesia', Annie Pohlman draws on studies of *testimonio* originating in Latin American studies. Her project explores narratives and silences about sexual violence that were perpetrated against women during the Indonesian killings of 1965-66 and the mass political detention of citizens under Suharto's New Order (1965-98). Pohlman's research attempts to gather and interpret the testimony of a generation of women that is rapidly diminishing, with their stories unheard. Here too the concept of trauma discourse is important: what strategies do these women use as a collective to describe - or not as the case may be - sexual violence and other human rights abuses under the New Order? How do they give witness, and find readers and listeners? Terri Tomsky's essay 'Fifty Years On: Melancholic (Re)collections and Women's Voices from the Partition of India' also takes up the legacy of historical trauma - in this case the partition of India and Pakistan in 1947-48. Tomsky is interested in a specific genre of trauma story about partition: the anthology, which has emerged as a major vehicle for the transmission of fictional and subsequently autobiographical narratives by and about women. Like *testimonio*, Tomsky suggests the anthology can play a critical role in developing a politics of collective trauma that can force an engagement with, in this case, the horrors of partition. These played out particularly on the bodies of women, and Tomsky engages with psychoanalytic readings that suggest the mourning of partition's victims and the working through of its violences have yet to be achieved.

In Pohlman's careful analysis of *testimonio* the sites of telling are critically important in the staging and documentation of trauma story. A similar point emerges differently in Jane Haladay's article '"I Must Know": Re-membering Native Women in the CAVNET_IW Community'. From some perspectives Haladay's study could scarcely be more different to Pohlman's: she is discussing new media, specifically a US-based internet community 'Communities Against Violence Network - Indigenous Women'. But like Pohlman, Haladay is concerned to understand how traumatic narratives about sexual violence that affects a specific female community – Native/American Indian, First Nations and Alaska Native women - can circulate and be heard, and why the sites of telling are so important. In trauma studies the concept of witnessing life story is critical: how are traumatic events perceived and received? As a potent 'site of telling', the internet community can receive and in turn deploy trauma story, but it cannot secure its reception. In her discussion of CAVNET_IW, Haladay examines a case study where objections are raised to the circulation of trauma story even amongst this compassionate collective. This raises issues of secondary witnessing, where exposure to trauma narratives of violence against women is itself experienced as traumatic. In return, issues about responsibility to the dead to both witness and honour their trauma suggest an ethical imperative to continue to read and respond to these postings. Here issues of ethics and responsibility that recur in trauma studies emerge as critical to examining everyday practices and engagement when new media is used as a site of telling and remembrance.

For Peter Read and Marivic Wyndham, both heritage historians, 'sites' are also critically important in the circulation of trauma story, yet in their chapter 'Putting Site Back into Trauma Studies' space is not virtual (as for Haladay) or *mise en scène* (as for Pohlman) but material and monumental. Read and Wyndham examine five sites of state violence in Santiago, Chile, to argue that place has a vitally important role to play in individual and collective healing following the brutality of the Pinochet regime, installed after the overthrow of the Allende government in 1973. As we have seen, the notion that trauma is ultimately unspeakable, beyond representation, recurs in trauma studies; against this, Read and Wyndham insist on the importance of sites of memorialisation, on the preservation of sites of torture, disappearance and detention for future generations and processes of healing.

The next chapters circle around the traumatic story that has in no small part been established through Peter Read's insistence on the power of testimony and witnessing the Stolen Generations. The question of how we are ourselves incorporated into processes of giving testimony and/or giving witness in the place of 'the second person' is an important one (see Whitlock, 'In the Second Person'; 'Becoming Migaloo'). For most contemporary Australian academics and writers of life narrative, indigenous and non-indigenous, the experience of witnessing Stolen Generations testimony a decade ago has been seminal to subsequent research and writing. In 'Textual Traumata: Letters to Lindy Chamberlain from the Australian Public', Deborah Staines explores the embedded repetition of trauma and guilt around issues of parenting and responsibility in her exploration of the Chamberlain archive. Lindy Chamberlain was tried and convicted of infanticide in 1980, and was incarcerated in Berrima jail despite her insistence that a dingo took her baby daughter Azaria. Subsequently released and exonerated, Chamberlain's case is paradigmatic in studies of contemporary Australian culture and society. Staines examines how the ripples of this story circled out to be experienced as a collective trauma, using as evidence selections from the 20,000 letters from the public to Chamberlain. Here, over a decade before the Stolen Generations testimony, empathic responses to the disappearance of Azaria stage an uncanny prequel to the later event. Issues of maternity and estrangement recur in Rosanne Kennedy's essay 'Defamiliarising the Maternal Trope: Assimilation and Estrangement in Holocaust "Hidden Children" and Stolen Generations Memoirs'. Like Staines, Kennedy is concerned to explore the traumatic legacies of abandonment and genocide, the Holocaust and the Stolen Generations. In a comparative reading of Sarah Kofman's memoir *Rue Ordener, Rue Labat* and Doris Pilkington's *Follow the Rabbit-Proof Fence*, an example of the comparative and expansive scholarship she called for in the introduction to *World Memory*, Kennedy examines how maternal tropes are deployed to authorise and naturalise ongoing and traumatic processes of dispossession in contemporary Australia. Now, as before, Australians witness interventions into indigenous communities 'in all innocence' rather than in complicity.

The final three chapters focus specifically on testimony in the wake of 9/11. Gillian Whitlock's article examines the exchange of letters between asylum seekers held on Nauru as part of the 'Pacific Solution', adopted by the Australian government in 2001, and the activists in Australia who vigorously campaigned on their behalf. These letters are just now beginning to become available to researchers, and Whitlock argues that they set some new agendas for scholarly research on the letters. Following this, in 'Hostile Witness: Torture Testimony in the War on Terror', Nina Philadelphoff-Puren takes up the question of how trauma story travels after 9/11 in a discourse analysis of the torture testimonies of two Guantanamo Bay detainees, Mamdouh Habib and David Hicks. Here testimony is rendered 'unspeakable', due not only to the devastating effects of trauma on the mind and body of the individual but also as a result of the attack on the detainees' ability to narrate at the level of rhetoric and the law. Finally, in 'From Grief to Grievance: Ethics and Politics in the Testimony of Anti-War Mothers', Cynthia Franklin and Laura Lyons examine the spaces to speak of the traumatic loss of mothers in the USA as a result of the Iraq war. As with Hicks and Habib, we can discern distinctive registers for recognising testimonial speech about grief and loss in the wake of the Iraq conflict, and at the same time it is equally apparent that other testimonies are rendered unspeakable. By contrasting the expressions of maternal grief and associated activist campaigns by Cindy Sheehan and Celeste Zappala, Franklin and Lyons discern the different rhetorical registers for testimony now, and the various uses of grief narrative in debates about Iraq and the 'war on terror'.

While these chapters draw on existing trauma theory, in each case they adapt and augment existing scholarship to meet the demands of taking key issues and concepts in trauma studies into global networks. Most obviously 'global' translates into an attention to life writing in what might be conceived of as 'postcolonial' worlds, and the legacies of old and new imperialisms. However it is also apparent that these contexts and the transnational passages of life writing require adaptation of key concepts in scholarly work on testimony and witnessing, for example, and also the incorporation of an expanded repertoire of texts and media. In *Trauma Texts* we set out to map the routes of what is now travelling theory.

References

Bennett, Jill and Rosanne Kennedy. *World Memory. Personal Trajectories in Global Time.* London: Palgrave Macmillan, 2003.

Caruth, Cathy. *Unclaimed Experience: Trauma, Narrative and History.* Baltimore: The Johns Hopkins UP, 1996.

Cvetkovich, Ann. *An Archive of Feelings. Trauma, Sexuality and Lesbian Public Cultures.* Durham and London: Duke UP, 2003.

Douglass, Ana and Thomas A. Vogler, eds. *Witness and Memory. The Discourse of Trauma.* New York and London: Routledge, 2003.

Felman, Shoshana and Dori Laub. *Testimony: Crises of Witnessing in Literature, Psychoanalysis, and History.* New York and London: Routledge, 1992.

Gilmore, Leigh. *The Limits of Autobiography: Trauma and Testimony.* Ithaca, NY: Cornell UP, 2001.

Kaplan, E. Ann. *Trauma Culture: The Politics of Terror and Loss in Media and Literature.* New Brunswick, New Jersey and London: Rutgers UP, 2005.

LaCapra, Dominick. *Representing the Holocaust: History, Theory, Trauma.* Ithaca, NY: Cornell UP, 1994.

Leys, Ruth. *Trauma: A Genealogy.* Chicago and London: The U of Chicago P, 2000.

Miller, Nancy K. and Jason Tougaw, eds. *Extremities. Trauma, Testimony and the Community.* Urbana and Chicago: U of Illinois P, 2002.

Oliver, Kelly. *Witnessing: Beyond Recognition.* Minneapolis and London: U of Minnesota P, 2001.

Read, Peter. *A Rape of the Soul So Profound: The Return of the Stolen Generation.* St Leonards: Allen and Unwin, 1999.

Sanders, Mark. *Ambiguities of Witnessing: Law and Literature in the Time of a Truth Commission.* Stanford, CA: Stanford UP, 2007.

Schaffer, Kay and Sidonie Smith. *Human Rights and Narrated Lives: The Ethics of Recognition.* New York: Palgrave Macmillan, 2006.

Whitlock, Gillian. 'In the Second Person: Narrative Transactions in Stolen Generation Testimony.' *Biography: An Interdisciplinary Quarterley* 24.1 (2001): 197–214.

— 'Becoming Migloo.' *The Ideas Market: An Alternative Take on Australia's Intellectual Life.* Ed. David Carter. Melbourne: Melbourne UP. 2001. 236559

— *Soft Weapons: Autobiography in Transit.* Chicago: U of Chicago P, 2007.

Yaeger, Patricia. 'Consuming Trauma; or, The Pleasures of Merely Circulating.' *Extremities. Trauma, Testimony and the Community.* Nancy K. Miller and Jason Tougaw, eds. Urbana and Chicago: U of Illinois P, 2002. 25–51.

A Transnational Hip Hop Nation: praCh, Cambodia, and Memorialising the Killing Fields

Cathy J. Schlund-Vials

Within Asian American Studies, the Cambodian American experience occupies a similar, yet by no means identical, discursive position as that of Holocaust survivors within Jewish and Jewish American cultural production. Cambodian American cultural production is shaped by a period of time widely known as 'the Killing Fields', an era dominated by the horrific policies enacted by Pol Pot and the communist Khmer Rouge. Between 1975 and 1979, approximately two million Cambodians perished due to execution, starvation, disease, and forced labour. This number represents 15 to 25 per cent of the contemporary Cambodian population. The memory of this genocide, along with the documentation of it, is the primary referent for the Cambodian American identity within the United States. It has been documented cinematically in the 1984

Academy-Award-winning film, *The Killing Fields*, which is arguably the most well-known cultural production about the genocide.

But *The Killing Fields* is not the only narrative about the genocide. In 2000, during the Cambodian New Year celebrations in Long Beach, California, Cambodian American rapper praCh distributed *Dalama: The End'n Is Just the Beginnin'*, a hip hop CD produced not in the studio but in his parents' garage.[1] praCh sampled Khmer Rouge propaganda speeches, rapped in English and Khmer, and based his lyrics on stories told to him by family members who had survived the Killing Fields.[2] The album featured members of Northstar Resurrec, a hip hop group begun in 1996 which included praCh and other Cambodian American rappers sparC da Polar, doZer, and Toeum Tom Chan.[3] A hip hop memoir, *Dalama: The End'n Is Just the Beginnin'* was by no means a financial success in the United States. In Cambodia, however, praCh was a phenomenon. Unbeknownst to the rapper, a copy of his CD made its way to Cambodia, was played on Phnom Penh radio, and its popularity increased through bootleg copies.[4] Renamed *Khmer Rouge Rap*, praCh's work was incredibly popular among Khmer youth, who connected with lyrics about the Cambodian genocide and Cambodian American life after the Killing Fields.[5] Although praCh had not been back to his homeland since he was a toddler, he became the number-one music artist in Cambodia.

Unintentionally, praCh created a transnational hip hop nation through his music, connecting Cambodian American and Khmer youth cultures. This connection is the entry point for this essay, which examines how Cambodian American youth memorialise the Killing Fields in a manner that is transnational and diasporically specific to the refugee experience. *Dalama: The End'n Is Just The Beginnin'* is the initial album in a trilogy, followed by *Dalama: The Lost Chapter* (2002). The primary title 'dalama' reflects praCh's desire to autobiographically combine drama and trauma, and he 'made up his own word and turned that into the story of his life' (May 77). The final album in the trilogy, *Dalama: Memoirs of an Invisible War*, is according to praCh, 'a very dark album ... about political turmoil', and is slated for release in April 2008 (May 81).

Focusing on praCh's second album, *Dalama: The Lost Chapter* (hereafter *The Lost Chapter*), I assert the rapper, through the interdisciplinary idiom of hip hop, negotiates individual, familial, and communal stories grounded in Cambodian refugee and Cambodian American experiences.[6] The four basic elements of the form—djaying, mcing (rapping), breakdancing, and graffiti—are auditory and visual signifiers of identity and location. Fundamental to hip hop is its potential to serve as a site of wisdom and a space of knowledge.[7] In praCh's work, knowledge takes the form of a genocidal history consistently relegated to the margins. However, praCh's role as knowledge producer goes beyond the reclamation of history. This reclamation intersects with a contemplation of how this history continues to impact a generation who are 'children of the Killing Fields' living in the United States.[8]

Identity and location—dominant themes in hip hop—are complicated with regard to the transnational Cambodian American refugee experience, which is problematised given US foreign policy in Southeast Asia during the Vietnam War.

US bombings of the Cambodian countryside destabilised an already fragile postcolonial government, paving the way for the Khmer Rouge takeover of Phnom Penh, which signalled the start of the Cambodian genocide. For the Cambodian American refugee subject, the United States is a paradoxical site responsible for dislocation from the country of origin yet it also serves as a significant place of refuge. Although Cambodian refugees have not exclusively relocated to the United States, aforementioned political actualities make the United States a potentially provocative space for examination. Furthermore, the passage of the 1980 Refugee Act facilitated the migration of over 100,000 Cambodian refugees to the United States. One of the largest Cambodian refugee communities is in Long Beach, California, which incidentally is praCh's home location. Cambodian American citizenship, circumscribed by particular dominant ethno-racial logics, US foreign policy, and US domestic policy, raises the question not only American identity, but also what it means to be Cambodian and Cambodian American in light of a genocidal history.

The memory of genocide is undeniably traumatic. Acts and projects of memorialisation attempt to negotiate trauma through remembrance and reconciliation. The negotiation of trauma through this two-sided process characterises praCh's hip hop project. praCh memorialises the Killing Fields in his work, and this memorialisation is geographically and culturally located in the United States and Cambodia. As the history of Cambodian memorialisation efforts (or rather, lack thereof) illustrates, praCh's albums engage contemporary issues of Cambodian selfhood and nationhood. Moreover, praCh's hip hop project, domestically produced and globally consumed, embodies what this issue's editors Gillian Whitlock and Kate Douglas suggest is a relatively under-examined and unexplored transit of testimony. The notion of transit—connotative of a journey or passing—is literally apparent in the global migration of praCh's debut album from Long Beach, California to Phnom Penh, Cambodia. This concept characterises the transits or journeys embedded in praCh's artistic project. *The Lost Chapter* thematically and artistically highlights Cambodian genocidal history, foregrounds the impact of this history on Cambodian American refugees, and recuperates Khmer artistic forms largely destroyed during the Khmer Rouge reign.

The memory of the Killing Fields and its legacy haunts *The Lost Chapter*. The genocide gives rise to multiple forms of traumatic memory within the narrative fabric of the album; images of death coexist with repeated directives to remember that past. The song, 'Stories', is emblematic of this negotiation. Its early placement in the album (as the second track) and chorus illustrate the album's central historical focus: 'Stories told by our parents to us/Before we go to bed about the field revolution/and two millions that are dead/Is in our head/ And it's hard to let go/but instead-a shedding tears/we're here to let you know/ about the Killing Fields/not long ago' (*The Lost Chapter*). praCh's lyrics emphasise the source of the traumatic story—'our parents'—directly referencing the Killing Fields and its human cost. The use of collective pronouns establishes that the auditory narrative which follows, rooted in the trauma of the genocide, is familial and communal. The temporal frame suggested—that the genocide did not happen 'long ago'—reminds the listener of the contemporary and historically relevant nature of praCh's narrative. praCh's lyrics highlight a more active subject position not predicated on 'shedding tears' but instead marked by the assertion that 'we're here to let you know ... about the Killing Fields'. Thus, the revelation of this genocidal history through testimony is cast as an act of power and agency.

With a total of twenty-one tracks, *The Lost Chapter* uses samples from American and Cambodian films, documentaries about the Killing Fields, and political speeches, including the address given by President George W. Bush following the 11 September attacks.[9] The majority of the compositions are in English, yet certain tracks feature Khmer and other pieces are bilingual (Khmer and English). In addition to compositions that privilege praCh as the primary mc, Cambodian American rappers and fellow Northstar Resurrec members doZer, Toeum Tom Chan, and sparC da Polar headline four tracks. Selected beats and background vocals are provided by the Universal Speakers, a pan-Southeast Asian American female trio.[10] praCh's father, Seng Ly, who speaks in Khmer, is also included in the album. Ho C. Chan, a pin peat musician living in the United States, figures keenly in the album's audioscape. Thus, praCh's *The Lost Chapter* is a polyvocal and intergenerational production very much embedded in familial and communal Cambodian/Cambodian American frameworks.[11] The inclusion of this polyvocal sensibility echoes one of the founding principles of hip hop as a form inextricably linked to community awareness and engagement.

This polyvocal sensibility, a multidisciplinary fusion of Khmer and US musical traditions, is politically significant to Cambodian genocidal history. For example, pin peat is a traditional Khmer music style that includes three singers, two bamboo xylophones, a flute, suspended brass pots, a two-headed drum, a large kettle drum, and a quadruple-reed instrument.[12] Based in Indian and Javanese traditions, Cambodian pin peat emerged during the Angkor era (c.842–c.1431 A.D.). It was revived as a music form during the twentieth century and was a cultural staple of the Khmer royal court. Pin peat also accompanied Cambodian Buddhist religious ceremonies. The form, along with classical Khmer ballet and Buddhism, was outlawed during the period of Democratic Kampuchea. Artists and religious practitioners were executed as part of the Khmer Rouge strategy to return the nation to 'year zero' through cultural, religious, and political obliteration.

Traditional Khmer music and dance artists were viewed as enemies of the communist Democratic Kampuchea state because of their affiliation to Prince Norodom Sihanouk and the Khmer royal court:[13]

> [During the period of Democratic Kampuchea], the new regime changed the country's name ... and sought zealously to eradicate all remnants of what they saw as a corrupt, feudal past. In order to murder the old culture they destroyed books, and musical instruments. ... As a revered symbol of Khmer culture, the musicians and dancers of the Royal Ballet were singled out by the new regime for

> elimination. They buried some instruments, costumes, and masks, and tried to escape detection by pretending to be workers in the rice fields. A few survived this way; most were put to death. ('America Provides Refuge' 37)

The obliteration of traditional Khmer art forms was thus related to a larger, nationally-sponsored project of erasure. The inclusion of pin peat as a musical foundation in praCh's *The Lost Chapter* is significant given its connection to the genocide. Such inclusion reflects a conscious attempt by the rapper to revive the tradition and create a markedly different Cambodian American hip hop form.[14] Most importantly, the focus on pin peat music in *The Lost Chapter* connects to a culturally-specific and pre-genocide Khmer identity. Concomitantly, praCh's use of pin peat challenges the Khmer Rouge intent to erase the past. This challenge is apparent in the instrumental composition, 'Pin Peat's Resurrection', which showcases pin peat master artist Ho C. Chan. The title of the track suggests the form's reemergence and continued livelihood, yet it also reads metaphorically as a marker of Khmer identity and culture. Simultaneously, the 'resurrection' suggests the agency of the Cambodian/Cambodian American to reconstruct a sense of selfhood in the face of overwhelming genocidal obliteration.

praCh supplements his use of traditional Khmer cultural forms with the improvisational theatrical form ayai. In ayai, one singer poses a question or rhyme, and the other singer responds in kind. The second singer typically answers with the last line sung. praCh maintains,

> Ayai is sort of like rap music, but in a Cambodian way. Ayai is like one poetry master to another poetry master going out on stage or in front of a village and competing with their wisdom, their knowledge about certain subjects, like their land, but it has to continuously rhyme. So basically—rap. Not all rap is about streets and drugs and partying. There's every variety of rap. With Cambodian ayai, it's sort of like that too. (May 80–81)

Traditionally accompanied by musicians, ayai can also be sung acappella. In *The Lost Chapter*, ayai echoes the tenets of rap, which is predicated on rhymes and repetition. praCh foregrounds ayai in the composition entitled, 'refleXion', spoken in Khmer. Alongside pin peat, the appearance of ayai within the album's Cambodian/Cambodian American imaginary reinforces the transnational nature of *The Lost Chapter*. This style is analogous to pin peat with regard to cultural reclamation and memory, and functions as yet another marker of Cambodian/Cambodian American selfhood and agency.

The artistic fusion of multiple music forms within the auditory imaginary of *The Lost Chapter* collapses multiple sociopolitical identities within the creative space of the album. National, familial, and individual traumatic narratives are embedded within the narrative framework of the album. The album's structure reflects the traumatic history of Cambodian refugees and Cambodian Americans in that it is organised chronologically from past to present. Historically, the initial compositions address the Khmer Rouge takeover of Phnom Penh (1975); the album's setting then shifts to 1979, the year of praCh's birth.

The remaining pieces, which reference 11 September and the PATRIOT Act, are, for the most part, located in the present.[15]

Structurally, the album is divided into three primary sections, including an intro (subtitled 'invasion'), an intermission ('RULES ...'), and an 'outro' ('p e a C e') (*The Lost Chapter*). *The Lost Chapter* begins with a brief traditional flute composition that is interrupted with an excerpt from the film, *The Killing Fields*. The cinematic sample is taken from a conversation between an American reporter, a member of the US military, a Cambodian soldier, and a Cambodian interpreter.[16] This scene concludes with an explosion, establishing for the listener Cambodia's war-torn landscape prior to the period of the Killing Fields. Entitled, 'Invasion', the sample takes the listener to 1975, presumably days before the Khmer Rouge takeover of Phnom Penh. The cinematic sample is followed by a second hip hop introduction featuring rapper doZer, who, in the midst of an electronic baseline, starts the aforementioned 'Stories' with a detailed account of Khmer Rouge occupation and subsequent evacuation of Phnom Penh. This account reveals national history, highlights familial anecdotes of disruption, and stresses individual trauma (subjects faced with incredible violence and under constant fear of death). The inclusion of a multimedia format—which combines samples from cinema, hip hop compositions, and traditional Khmer music—is replicated throughout the album.

Next, the album moves to an excerpt from the documentary, *Year Zero: The Silent Death of Cambodia* (1979), narrated by Australian journalist and documentary filmmaker John Pilger.[17] praCh interrupts the documentary narrative with a rap about the political landscape of Democratic Kampuchea in a song entitled, 'Power, Territory, and Rice'. praCh recounts the evacuation of Phnom Penh through a hip hop narrative, providing another lens through which to consider Cambodian national history. In the chorus, praCh connects the evacuation to a larger political agenda which includes war, destabilisation, and power, along with its inevitable cost: 'It's about Power, Territory, and Rice,/And of course that comes with a hefty price./Whenever there's war, there's always sacrifice, /And it's usually the innocent who lose their life' (*The Lost Chapter*).

Furthermore, praCh examines in 'Power, Territory, and Rice' the generational impact of the Killing Fields, asserting, 'No one was told who was running the country but ah,/Only that those in power was called "Angka"./Children's was brainwash into believing in them,/They was taught that: "there's no such thing as parents"' (*The Lost Chapter*). The focus on children and erasure is relevant to contemporary Khmer youth, who, as the reception of praCh's first album illustrates, have little to no knowledge of the Killing Fields. Moreover, Cambodian American cultural production is largely characterised by a resistance to forget the past despite the Khmer Rouge directive to disremember, reinforced by the lack of sustained memorialisation efforts in contemporary Cambodia.

The Lost Chapter's subsequent pieces enumerate the experiences of Cambodians during the time of the Killing Fields. For example, track six, entitled 'The Great Escape', focuses on praCh's familial story of flight. After 'The Great Escape', the album shifts to a more contemporary contemplation of the

Cambodian refugee and the Cambodian American in the United States. Nonetheless, this contemplation—which for the most part dominates the remaining fifteen tracks of *The Lost Chapter*—explicitly and implicitly references the initial history of the Killing Fields. This connection is manifest in direct mentions to the Killing Fields and is suggested in the use of Khmer as a significant linguistic foundation in the album. Repeatedly, praCh's compositions stress national and familial history, Khmer culture, and Cambodian American identity.

The auditory elements of the album are visually replicated in praCh's album cover, which features Cambodian architecture, an American cityscape, and a ship. Together, these images signify the journey from Cambodia to the United States, reminding the listener of the transnational experience of the rapper. Given the communal stresses in the album's lyrics and artistic collaborations, the images reflect a larger Cambodian/Cambodian American migration history. praCh is also mindful of individual history, apparent in two other images that appear on the album's cover—a tree and a hut. These two images are significant given the location of praCh's birth. According to the rapper, in 1979 '... my mom was pregnant with me. She had me in a hut. Later, my parents went back to Cambodia and videotaped the tree I was born under, but the hut's no longer there' (May 73). This birth location is confirmed in the previously mentioned 'The Great Escape', which opens with the assertion that praCh 'was born in a hut/umbilical cord cut' (*The Lost Chapter*).

The revelation of praCh's origins quickly gives way to the trauma which accompanies the Cambodian subject who attempts to cross into the Thai border. The composition, which includes an almost violin-like backbeat, implicitly stresses the drama of the situation and reminds the listener of the danger this journey entails. This danger is confirmed lyrically in the chorus, when praCh states, 'watch out!/for boobie traps and land mines,/ain't no time to take breaks,/death is close behind,/night or day it's not OK!/gotta stay awake!/no matter what it takes,/we gotta make/the Great Escape!' (*The Lost Chapter*). The refugee subject is cast in a manner that acknowledges the trauma of 'the great escape' while simultaneously highlighting the degree to which this same Cambodian subject is empowered precisely because of the struggle. praCh asserts,

> when there [is] total silence,/you know danger ahead./and when the bomb goes off/then you know someone is dead./but forward ahead./we gotta make it further./no matter what it takes/we gotta make it across the border./we lost our heart, but found the strength in our soul,/words can't describe,/but the stories must be told./the fields, the jungles,/the mountains of death./the struggle continues,/but we're gonna make it! (*The Lost Chapter*)

The above excerpt suggests that, despite the loss of homeland and in the face of 'the mountains of death', the collective 'we'—in this case praCh's family—still finds strength that 'words can't describe' to enact 'the great escape'. This characterisation stresses a familial narrative and confirms the articulation of a

Cambodian agency embedded in a difficult, dangerous, and unimaginable journey to the border.

Moreover, in 'The Great Escape', praCh alludes to his own project, maintaining that 'stories must be told', and anticipates the next rap composition, entitled, 'I Just Want You to Understand'. This eighth track is preceded by 'Pin Peat's Resurrection'. Unlike previous tracks on *The Lost Chapter*, 'I Just Want You to Understand' combines, in the space of the composition, traditional Khmer music styles and hip hop. The song begins with a digitised pin peat beat and combines contemporary hip hop with traditional Khmer music. The pin peat beat is supplemented by an additional electronic bass line, reinforcing a transnational musical fusion between Khmer and American forms. The composition takes an autobiographical turn when praCh begins to rap. praCh states that he is:

> a messenger, a writer, inspired by the truth/take you behind the scenes like Fox 10 o'clock news/firsthand experience a living proof/100% special delivery to you/ when I first started off it was just for fun/now I'm doin' it cause they say it can't be done/I love narration tellin' my story that's my hobby/if money wasn't involved I'd probably do it for free/not for publicity or fame/cause all I want is for people to understand. (*The Lost Chapter*)

praCh enunciates a form of selfhood linked to his ability to provide the listener with a 'behind the scenes ... firsthand experience' embedded in a 'love of narration'. Most importantly, praCh's revelation of a significant historical truth through 'firsthand experience' facilitates a transit of testimony which allows Cambodian Americans to reclaim their past and continue as active agents in the present. This role of praCh as a cultural broker and knowledge producer is illustrated in the song's chorus, when the rapper maintains, 'I just want you to understand/it must be taught/history must be told/I just want you to understand/the past is unlocked/we played a key role' (*The Lost Chapter*). The emphasis on a collective 'we', coupled with a mention of a past 'unlocked', connects Cambodian/Cambodian American communal modalities to the official narrative of nationhood through history. Thus, praCh begins from an individualised position as a 'messenger of truth' who then connects his work to a larger Cambodian/Cambodian American sense of agency and selfhood.

Returning briefly to structure, it is admittedly difficult to divide the album into geographically or politically distinct sections. For example, the song, 'S-21 (Tuol Sleng)', about the infamous prison in Phnom Penh, is rendered in Khmer, and is placed rather late in the album (as the eighteenth track). Its placement, coupled with its linguistic characteristics, reminds the listener that the album is rooted in an ongoing contemplation of the Cambodian genocide. Concomitantly, with a piece entitled, 'TUES', which examines the attacks of 11 September, praCh blurs the lines between simplistic nation-state affiliations, claiming that he is both Khmer (Cambodian) *and* American. In this piece, praCh raps about the traumatic memory of 11 September. This composition reiterates in content and form to the album's reification of national identity through trauma. praCh articulates a transnational sensibility that traverses multiple borders and collapses the space between Cambodia and the United States.

Thus, praCh creates through the inclusion of traditional Cambodian music, samples from Khmer movies, *The Killing Fields*, and documentaries, and rhymes spoken in English and Khmer, a transnational Cambodian American subjectivity that resists a singular location in one geographic place or historical place. Instead, this subjectivity follows the trajectory of Cambodian American youth from the Killing Fields of Cambodia to the streets of Long Beach to the INS lines in a post-11 September United States. The culmination of this transnational trajectory is apparent in praCh's 'Art of Fact', a composition that combines artistically and thematically the album's primary motifs. What precedes this nineteenth track is the aforementioned rap about 'S-21', rendered in Khmer. What follows is a spoken portion entitled, 'out-tro', spoken in Khmer by Seng Ly, praCh's father, who states, 'We shouldn't argue about race. We are all one. We must learn to live together'. The inclusion of his father's voice reinforces the intergenerational transit of testimony within *The Lost Chapter*'s imaginary.

The transnational meditation on Cambodian/Cambodian American identity is confirmed in 'Art of Fact'. This contemplation is reflected in the fusion of Khmer and American music styles reminiscent of 'I Just Want You to Understand', and the song's initial instrumentation echoes that of a traditional pin peat flute. Further, its lyrics and rhythms suggest a fusion of Cambodian and Cambodian American identities. The piece blends R & B, a Cambodian pin peat beat, an electronic bass line, and a traditional Cambodian flute. praCh reminds the listener of his refugee past, beginning with the assertion that:

> Beyond the killing field,/a quarter of a century after the genocide./after 2 million people murdered,/the other 5 million survive/the fabric of the culture,/ beauty drips the texture,/I find myself in Long Beach,/the next Cambodian mecca. ... /here's a gap in our generation,/between the adults and kids,/but since I'm bilingual/I'ma use communication as a bridge. (*The Lost Chapter*)

praCh mentions the two million lost alongside the five million who survived, and the song stresses the need to communicate in order to reconcile the past. This sense of communication becomes intergenerationally significant with praCh's claim that he is 'bilingual', intent on, as the lyric continues, 'knock[ing] down the walls/between me and my parents', a subject who 'listens to their stories on all/without interference' (*The Lost Chapter*). praCh articulates a transnational location for Cambodian/Cambodian American identity through the declaration that he is in 'Long Beach ... the next Cambodian mecca' while underscoring a generation gap that prevents dialogue between 'adults and kids'. His assertion of bilingualism is a solution to this gap, and the song repeatedly returns to praCh's agency as a Cambodian American rapper.

Hence, praCh complicates this transnational solution with an acknowledgement of life in the United States, and the composition shifts to this particular location. Critical of 'the American Dream', praCh stresses the experience of

Cambodian American youth who must face 'terrorist and INS deportation' due to a US policy of 'one strike and you're out' (allusions to the 1996 Immigration Reform and the PATRIOT Act, which allowed for the deportation of 1,600 Cambodian/Cambodian Americans in 2001 and 2002) and gang life ('code of the streets'). praCh is not only critical of the promise of the United States as a place of possibility; he reminds the listener of the history of the Killing Fields. It is this history, reiterated throughout the album and throughout the song, which partially contextualises the experiences of Cambodian American youth. praCh includes a political critique of the United States; he then addresses generational tension and shifting family values ('fixing up marriages' and commodity fetishes in the form of 'fast cars'). This layering lyrically echoes the layering of musical texts, establishing the transnational and conflicted (at times conflicting) experiences of Cambodian American youth in the United States.

In a recent interview, praCh stated:

> Hip hop to me is the voice of the youth. Telling how one really feels about their way of living and how they are living. Their surrounding[s], their environment, or just one's story . . . It's not just talking into the mic, it's talking to the world. As for me growing up, it was all around me. Hip hop, rap, breakdancing, graffiti art. It's not just music, it's the culture I grew up in. But as an Asian, Cambodian, I had to tell my own story because no one else was going to tell it for me. Once I was able to record my voice I knew what I was going to say. I can only talk about what I know best. And that is my History. And my history is in my family and me. We lived and went through it.[18]

Within *The Lost Chapter*, praCh is the carrier of the Cambodian past and the embodiment of a Cambodian American who proudly maintains he is 'Khmer' and 'refuse[s] to let his culture die'. praCh provides an avenue of resistance through hip hop rooted in the past yet negotiates the present. His lyrics are matched by the transnational structure and content of the album with regard to language, culture, and tradition. praCh firmly articulates a Cambodian American subjectivity that uses, as the title of the song suggests, 'art' to address 'fact', creating, in the process, a memorial to the history and legacy Killing Fields and a monument to Cambodian American identity.

praCh's cultural work is more significant when contextualised against the lack of memorialisation in Cambodia and the paucity of such memorials in the United States. In Cambodia, the primary sites for memorialisation—Tuol Sleng (S-21) and Choeung Ek—were constructed during the Vietnamese occupation of Cambodia in the early 1980s. Paul Williams observes that although 'survivors of the DK [Democratic Kampuchea] regime have constructed seventy-eight genocide memorials in towns and rural districts', Tuol Sleng and Choeung Ek are the only two government-sanctioned sites that exist in the nation (247). These memorials privilege a politicised narrative of liberation, wherein the Khmer Rouge regime is cast as an enemy of the Vietnamese-liberated state. No culturally and politically-specific Cambodian space exists within such memorials. Nor is there space for a Cambodian narrative of the Killing Fields that problematises the potentially imperialistic position of the Vietnamese not as liberators but as occupiers. Because of the degree to which Cambodian cultural and political life was obliterated between 1975 and 1979, Cambodian funding for such memorials and the creation of these memorials is still not feasible.

After the 1988 Vietnamese withdrawal, the continued presence of the Khmer Rouge in sociopolitical realms prompted the Cambodian government to seek political reconciliation through a peace process. Cambodians were asked to forgive Khmer Rouge leaders and forget the genocide. In 1996, the Cambodian government emphasised national reconciliation. Upon making pledges of peace, former Khmer Rouge fighters were welcomed back into the Cambodian government. Three years after Pol Pot's death, in December 2001, Prime Minister Hun Sen called for the restoration of current memorials and the future memorialisation of other burial sites. Additionally, the prime minister called for the construction of a memorial museum that would facilitate a national reconciliation. However, the construction of such a museum has yet to occur. Just as there has been no nationally-sanctioned and funded memorial effort, no consistent policy for reconciliation exists in Cambodia.[19] This brief history of memorialisation efforts in Cambodia illustrates the weight which falls upon praCh and other Cambodian American cultural producers who negotiate the problematic past in their work.[20]

As a Cambodian American cultural producer, praCh creates a particular transnational transit of testimony, wherein the history of the Killing Fields travels across nation-state borders. praCh's work memorialises the genocide and generationally intersects with the work of other 1.5 generation Cambodian Americans ('1.5 generation Cambodian Americans' refers to those who were born in Cambodia but who left prior to their teens). It is this group who has recently taken on the task of memory work with regard to the Killing Fields. This memory work is largely literary and autobiographical, and such narratives are often written from the perspective of those who survived the Killing Fields as children.

The titles of three full-length autobiographies that have recently been published are illustrative: Buth Keo's *The Stones Cry Out: A Cambodian Childhood, 1975–1980* (originally published in 1986 and republished in 1999), Chanrithy Him's *When Broken Glass Floats: Growing Up Under the Khmer Rouge*, and Luong *Ung's First They Killed My Father: A Daughter of Cambodia Remembers*. Keo, Him, and Ung each begin with a brief account of life before 1975 (the year the Khmer Rouge came to power), recount life under the Khmer Rouge, and examine life after the Khmer Rouge (usually from the position of a refugee in a camp or in the United States). The narrative emphasis of each work revolves around coming of age under the regime of the Khmer Rouge.

The impulse to memorialise Cambodian history connects praCh's work to that of other Cambodian American cultural producers who transnationally re-imagine Cambodian nationhood and selfhood.[21] Unlike praCh, these authors do not explicitly focus on the journey from Southeast Asia to the United States, nor is there a sustained exploration of Cambodian American identity. Rather, the narrative is located primarily in Cambodia, and the focus is not on Cambodian

American but Cambodian subjectivity and selfhood. Despite the overwhelming presence of the genocide as a historical, social, and political foundation in *The Lost Chapter*, praCh also emphasises Cambodian American identity, artistically mapping the journey from traumatised subject to empowered agent. It is the multisided contemplation of Cambodian/Cambodian American identity—wherein praCh is a child of the Killing Fields and a product of an American upbringing—which signals a particularly Cambodian American transit of testimony between Cambodia and the United States. The memorialisation of the Cambodian genocide exists alongside articulations of a Cambodian American who must, because of sociopolitical actualities, re-imagine the country of his birth from the country of settlement.

Thus, praCh's hip hop exploration of Cambodian American subjectivity through a double-sided resistance against erasure and marginalisation disrupts the 'traditional' Killing Fields narrative largely set in Cambodia and Southeast Asia. Furthermore, the degree to which praCh focuses his hip hop project on questions of empowerment, assertions of ethnic pride, and critiques of policies that in fact target Cambodian American youth signal a significant departure from other 1.5 generation Cambodian American literary productions. The multiple forms of testimony in *The Lost Chapter*—wherein Cambodian history and culture are mediated in the same artistic space of Cambodian American experience and culture—force a transnational consideration of trauma connected to Cambodian and Cambodian American identity. *The Lost Chapter* militates against essentialised contemplations of unilateral selfhood, problematises notions of belonging, and revises conceptualisations of nationhood.

In conclusion, politics of representation—including questions of authenticity, notions of narrative authority, and ideas of what constitutes a 'valid' Cambodian selfhood—are vital to scholarly examinations of Cambodian/Cambodian American cultural work in which political, social, and personal affiliations are imagined *vis-à-vis* the genocide, supporting a particular solidarity built on trauma and resistance. praCh's work complicates Killing Fields remembrance in that it explicitly negotiates the Cambodian past alongside the Cambodian American present. Additionally, praCh's *The Lost Chapter* functions as a transnational text in form and content, which is haunted by the trauma of the Killing Fields yet paradoxically uses this trauma as the basis for a Cambodian American form of selfhood linked to resistance and remembrance. Nonetheless, praCh's project is also linked to other Cambodian American cultural producers who consistently return to memorialisation as a thematic focus in their work. Such memorialisation and the negotiation of trauma intersect with constructions of nationhood and contestations over national memory. Ernest Renan's notion of historical amnesia, fundamental to nation-building in the twentieth and twenty-first centuries, is relevant to a post-genocide Cambodian nationalism that liminally exists between memory and erasure.[22] And, within Cambodian American cultural production, impulses to remember coexist with desires to never forget.

Notes

[1] 'praCh' is the stage name for Prach Ly. For the remainder of this essay I will refer to the rapper by his stage name. According to praCh, 'The meaning of *praCh* is "advisor to the king" or "person who talks a lot". But my parents didn't name me praCh because of that. The area where I was born was called Veal Srae K'rach: farmland of K'prach ... They [his parents] didn't know what to name me when I was born at the camp place, so they just named me praCh' (May 73). The 'C' in 'praCh' is capitalised to emphasise the rapper's connection to his Cambodian roots. praCh was born in 1979 near Battambang, Cambodia. For consistency, I will use the following spelling: 'hip hop'.

[2] For the debut album, praCh used a karaoke machine, microphones, and a tape player. CDs bought from local record stores provided the basis for beats and instrumentation on the album, and the album was produced in three months (May 77). Tracks in the debut album include: [1] 'Intro: The Temple of Peace—Takeover'; [2] 'The Letter (Prisoner of War)'; [3] 'Skit: Start Anew, Nuth'n Has Gone Before'; [4] 'The YearZero!'; [5] 'Interlude: Peak of Light'; [6] 'Welcome'; [7] 'Interlude: New Hope'; [8] 'Out-tro: The Burden of Power—The Countdown 3, 2, 1 ...'; [9] 'NorthSide (We High)' (featuring Toeum); [10] 'Walk-a-Block' (featuring Northstar Resurrec); [11] 'War on the Street'; [12] 'Knowledge, Nix-Mo'; [13] 'Ah-Ye (Khmer Rap!)'; [15] 'Make Money Take Money'; [16] 'Zip (Da N Nite)' (featuring doZer and Pinner); and [17] 'Take Your Time'. praCh's second album, *Dalama: The Lost Chapter*, utilises a similar structure with regard to sections.

[3] According to *Khmer Connection* reviewer Poli Bou, praCh was the first Cambodian American rapper to complete a full-length hip hop album. Bou provides a useful overview and comprehensive summary of praCh's *Dalama: The End'n Is Just The Beginnin'*.

[4] Although unsure as to who transported the album from Long Beach, California to Phnom Penh, Cambodia, praCh suggested in a 2003 interview that 'DJ Sop, a well-known deejay in Cambodia' was at the 2000 Cambodian New Year celebration and may have been responsible for its play on Cambodian radio (May 78).

[5] According to praCh, in the Cambodian reproduction, 'The cover was gone. The artwork was gone. My name was gone. The credits were gone. Gone out the window' (May 79). It was not until the rapper was contacted by Gina Chon, a reporter for *Asiaweek* and *Cambodian Daily*, that praCh was aware of his success abroad. Shortly after Chon's story was published in *Asiaweek*, praCh's work was featured in periodicals including the *Los Angeles Times*, *Newsweek*, and the *New York Post*. He was the focus of the American television program, *Frontline*, and interviewed in the American radio broadcast, *Voice of America*. I mention these publications and shows because they are referenced in praCh's song, 'I Just Want You to Understand', from his second album.

[6] Although the debut album is certainly of interest with regard to its distribution history, and lyrically adheres to praCh's larger goal to memorialise the Killing Fields in his work, this initial production relies heavily on other artists' work for instrumentation and beat. *The Lost Chapter* is more original production with regard to instrumentation and beat production. As praCh maintains,

> I think *Dalama Two* is more—I don't want to say creative, but I gave it its own life. It's not a duplication of the first album. It bears a similarity because it's an autobiography too. But at the same time, it holds its own ground. I mixed Cambodian traditional music with rap; I created a

> Cambodian hip-hop beat. And this time, I was really proud to say, all the beats and instrumentals were ours. (May 80)

The Lost Chapter allows for a more multidisciplinary consideration of Cambodian American hip hop that accommodates an examination of lyrics and music.

[7] Hip hop, as an interdisciplinary form of resistance, has not escaped scholarly attention within the United States. Jeff Chang and Nitasha Sharma have written extensively and provocatively about hip hop as a form in which to examine racial and ethnic construction. Chang's *Can't Stop, Won't Stop* is a useful introduction to the history of the form from the 1970s to the present. Sharma's work examines hip hop through a comparative ethno-racial frame that brings together African American and South Asian American cultural producers. S. Craig Watkins's text, *Hip Hop Matters* highlights the contradictory nature of hip hop as a terrain of commodification and a significant site of resistance. Other useful examinations of the form include Tricia Rose's *Black Noise: Rap Music and Black Culture in Contemporary America*; *Droppin' Science: Critical Essays on Rap Music and Hip Hop Culture* by William Eric Perkins; Russell A. Potter's *Spectacular Vernaculars: Hip Hop and the Politics of Postmodernism*; and *The 'Hood Comes First: Race, Space, and Place in Rap and Hip-Hop* by Murray Forman.

[8] 'Children of the Killing Fields' is a line from praCh's 'Resurrect' on his debut album.

[9] What follows is an ordered listing of the nineteen tracks which constitute *Dalama: The Lost Chapter*: [1] intro ('invasion'); [2] 'STORIES' (featuring doZer); [3] skits, 'the YearZero and One' (documentary sample); [4] 'Power, Territory, and Rice'; [5] skits, 'the aftermath' (documentary sample); [6] 'The Great Escape!'; [7] 'Pin Peat's Resurrection' (featuring Khmer traditional musician Ho C. Chan); [8] 'I Just Want You to Understand!'; [9] 'D'eBreeZZe' (featuring sparC da Polar); [10] 'Min-Tom-le-Da'; [11] 'Sox-Si-Bie'; [12] 'intermission' (RULES ...); [13] 'refleXtion'; [14] 'Wisc's That'; [15] 'Neutral (before the war)'; [16] 'Tues'; [17] 's.i.c.'; [18] 'S-21' (tuol sleng); [19] 'Art of Fact'; [20] 'out-tro', and [21] ('p e a C e').

[10] According to www.muestic.com, the Universal Speakers, who include Cambodian American, Laotian American, and Thai American female singers, combine reggae, hip hop, and R&B in their music (accessed 3 May 2007).

[11] The inclusion of Ho C. Chan is of particular note because of his connection to traditional Khmer music (pin peat).

[12] The Khmer names for the instruments enumerated are as follows: *reneat* (bamboo xylophones), *gong vong* (brass pots), *kloy* (flute), *sampho* (two-headed drum), *skor thom* (a large kettle drum), and *srlai* (the oboe-like instrument).

[13] Prince Sihanouk, following the death of his father in 1960, became the Cambodian head of state. In 1963, he forcibly changed the Cambodian constitution so that he would remain head of state for the remainder of his life. He was deposed in 1970 by then prime minister Lon Nol.

[14] In addition to his own work, praCh is also a music producer. Among his current projects is an album of traditional pin peat music. praCh asserts, 'I really want to help revive that. There are only about four Cambodian master musicians left in the United States, and Mr. Chan Ho [Ho Chan] is one of them. He plays all the instruments. I was privileged to have him play interludes on traditional instruments for *Dalama Two*. There's also some traditional music with me rapping over it; his son played that' (May 80).

[15] The USA PATRIOT Act (Uniting and Strengthening America by Providing Appropriate Tools Required to Intercept and Obstruct Terrorism Act of 2001) was passed following the 11 September 2001 attacks. A 342-page document, the act was linked to national, state, and local anti-terrorist initiatives. Much more can certainly be written with regard to the act's impact on civil liberties and law enforcement, but

what is most relevant is that the act reconfigured the authority of the Immigration and Nationality Service (INS) and was used to facilitate the deportation of individuals who had committed 'aggravated felonies'. Such felonies lacked concrete definition, and crimes that fell under this rubric ranged from writing bad checks to murder. 1,500 Cambodian/Cambodian Americans living in the United States were threatened with deportation, and this story is mentioned in praCh's 'Art of Fact'.

[16] *The Killing Fields*. The film was based on the experiences of Cambodian journalist Dith Pran during the period of the genocide. Dr. Haing S. Ngor portrayed Pran in the production, and won the American Academy-Award for Best Supporting Actor in 1985. Dr. Ngor died in a gang-related shooting in 1996.

[17] Pilger's film highlights the extent to which the genocide in Cambodia was met with indifference on the world stage by various governments. It includes interviews with survivors and footage of Cambodia during and after the period of the Killing Fields.

[18] Interview conducted 24 November 2006.

[19] The lack of a nationally-sanctioned memorial in Cambodia is reflected by the absence of justice for victims of the Killing Fields on the world stage. It was not until March 2003 that the United Nations reached a draft agreement with the Cambodian government for the formation of an international criminal tribunal to try former Khmer Rouge leaders. Such an effort occurred after five years of negotiation and twenty-four years after the Khmer Rouge were driven out of power. The rules for the tribunal were recently codified in March 2007. According to Ek Madra,

> Pol Pot, the 'Brother Number One' of the government which spawned the 'Killing Fields', died in 1998. But 'Brother Number Two' Nuon Chea, former head of state Khieu Samphan and ex-Foreign Minister Ieng Sary are all living free in Cambodia and are due to face trial. The only senior Khmer Rouge figure in detention is Duch, head of the notorious Tuol Sleng interrogation center, a former school in Phnom Penh where at least 14 000 people were tortured and executed before a Vietnamese invasion ended their rule in 1979. (*Reuters* 16 March 2007)

In August 2007, news that Duch would testify against the Khmer Rouge to a UN-backed international war crimes tribunal was released, and Nuon Chea was charged with war crimes.

[20] In the United States, the Khmer Institute and the Cambodian American Heritage Museum in Chicago have created virtual memorials to the Killing Fields. To draw briefly from James Young's work, these virtual sites, along with other cultural productions, provide the significant spaces 'where groups of people gather to create a common past for themselves' and construct 'constitutive narratives' (6).

[21] Marianne Hirsch's work on postmemory provides a useful entrée into a discussion of memory in 1.5 generation Cambodian American youth. Hirsch draws from the traumatic memory of the Holocaust and its continued position as a referent for familial memory for children of survivors. Hirsch asserts that postmemory 'characterises the experience of those who grow up dominated by narratives that preceded their birth, whose own belated stories are evacuated by the stories of the previous generation shaped by traumatic events that be neither understood nor recreated' (22). However, Cambodian American youth and their respective cultural productions do not fit neatly into Hirsch's rubric. Such productions reflect the experiences of those who, as children, lived during the genocide yet have left their country of origin prior to their teens. The narrative of the Killing Fields is one that is intimately linked to childhood remembrance.

[22] Renan, 'What is a Nation?'. Written at a time of shifting global dynamics and in light of large-scale colonial projects, Renan dismisses racial and linguistic foundations for nationhood. According to Renan,

> A nation is a soul, a spiritual principle. Two things, which in truth are one, constitute this soul or spiritual principle. One lies in the past, one in the present. One is the possession in common of a rich legacy of memories, the other is present-day consent, the desire to live together, the will to perpetuate the value of the heritage that one has received in individual form ... Where national memories are concerned, griefs are of more value than triumphs, for they impose duties and require a common effort. (52–53)

References

'America Provides Refuge for an Imperiled Art.' *Music Educators Journal* 69 May (1983): 37–38.

Bou, Poli. Rev. of *Dalama: The End'n Is Just The Beginnin'* 9 June 2000. *Khmer Connection.* 14 May 2007. <http:khmer.cc/channels/0,8,7,01,4438.html>.

Chang, Jeff. *Can't Stop, Won't Stop.* London: Ebury, 2005.

Forman, Murray. *The 'Hood Comes First: Race, Space, and Place in Rap and Hip-Hop.* Hanover, NH: Wesleyan UP, 2002.

Him, Chanrithy. *When Broken Glass Floats: Growing Up Under the Khmer Rouge.* New York: Norton, 2000.

Hirsch, Marianne. *Family Frames: Photography, Narrative, and Postmemory.* Boston, MA: Harvard UP, 1997.

Keo, Buth (Molyda Szymusiak). The Stones Cry Out: A Cambodian Childhood, 1975–1980. Tras. Jane Hamilton-Merritt and Linda Coverdale. New York, NY: Hill and Wang Publishing, 1986; Bloomington, ID: Indiana UP, 1999.

The Killing Fields. Dir. Roland Joffe. Perf. Sam Waterston, Haing S. Ngor, Spaulding Gray, Craig T. Nelson, and John Malkovitch. Enigma (First Casualty Ltd), 1984.

Madra, Ek. 'Khmer Rouge Trial Rules Agreed at Last.' *Reuters* 16 March 2007. Reuters 21 April 2007 <http://www.reuters.com/article/latestCrisis/idUSBKK21057>.

May, Sharon. Interview with praCh. 'Art of fact.' *Manoa* 16.1 (2004): 73–82.

praCh. *Dalama: The End'n Is Just the Beginnin'.* Long Beach, CA: Mujestic Records, 2000.

——. *Dalama: The Lost Chapter.* Long Beach, CA: Mujestic Records, 2002.

——. *Dalama: Memoirs of an Invisible War.* Forthcoming.

——. 'It's Not Just Muzix, It's a Movement.' 12 May 2007. <http://www.mujestic.com/p_r_a_c_h>

Perkins, William Eric. *Droppin' Science: Critical Essays on Rap Music and Hip Hop Culture.* Philadelphia: Temple UP, 1995.

Potter, Russell A. *Spectacular Vernaculars: Hip Hop and the Politics of Postmodernism.* Albany: State U of New York P, 1995.

Renan, Ernest. 'What is a Nation?' *Becoming National: A Reader.* New York: Oxford UP, 1996. 41–55.

Rose, Tricia. *Black Noise: Rap Music and Black Culture in Contemporary America.* Middletown, CT: Wesleyan UP, 1994.

Ung, Luong. *First They Killed My Father: A Daughter of Cambodia Remembers.* New York: HarperCollins, 2000.

Uniting and Strengthening America by Providing Appropriate Tools Required to Intercept and Obstruct Terrorism (USA PATRIOT ACT) Act of 2001. 26 October 2001. Pub. L. 107–56.

Watkins, S. Craig. *Hip Hop Matters*. Boston: Airlift, 2005.

Williams, Paul. 'Witnessing Genocide: Vigilance and Remembrance at Tuol Sleng and Choeung Ek.' *Holocaust and Genocide Studies* 18.2 (2004): 234–55.

Year Zero: The Silent Death of Cambodia. Dir. David Munro. Perf. John Pilger. Associated Television (ATV) Network Limited, 1979.

Young, James. *The Texture of Memory*. New Haven, CT: Yale UP, 1993.

Drawings by Tanzanian Street Youths

Markus Wiencke

This article focuses on my contact with children and youths who live on the streets in Mwanza—the second biggest city in Tanzania. It reflects upon their individual stories about the traumatic circumstances of their daily existence (Wiencke).[1] Mwanza, the capital of the region Mwanza, is situated in the northwest of Tanzania, sitting directly on the shores of Lake Victoria. Mwanza plays an important role in international trade, being a location of commerce for Uganda, Kenya, Rwanda, Democratic Republic of Congo, as well as within Tanzania. Many people live on the shores of Lake Victoria, making a living out of fishing, and a great number of companies there have specialised in processing and trading fish. The city's actual expanse is fairly large, although the city centre, with its shops and offices, is quite small.

Street children endure a life of traumatic and continuous violence and abuse. Many of the children no longer have any connection with their families, having been abandoned for various reasons. Faced with the immediate dangers and threatening nature of the streets, they have developed different coping strategies: working odd jobs, theft, begging and prostitution or they will sniff glue to get high and numb themselves to the pains of hunger and fear. At night they will sleep in doorways, under market stands, or—if they have found someone willing to support them—in small rooms.

The complex and descriptive concept of 'life world', which respects the subjective perceptions of the street children themselves, formed the framework of my research. How do children living on the streets experience their own situation? During fieldwork in the year 2001, I aimed to obtain close impressions and gain insights into the lives of my informants by means of ethnographic and problem-centred interviewing methods, drawings and by the use of participant-observation (Spradley; Witzel). The twenty-two informants were between thirteen and twenty-two years old; fifteen were male and seven female. The data thus obtained was subsequently analysed using content analysis (Mayring 2003). Following Geertz's example, I obtained 'thick descriptions' (24) of the life world of street children in Mwanza. Wolff (339–40) points out that research is always an intervention into a social system. According to this understanding, my presence as a researcher represented a disturbing factor to the street children, and it follows from this that questions of validity arise about to what extent my constructions originate in the constructions of the researched, and to what extent this origin is comprehensible to others. For this reason, I made the research process as comprehensible to others as possible by providing detailed documentation (cf. Matt).

The reality street children in Mwanza face can be approached using artwork made by children and youths who live on the streets. These drawings enrich our understanding of the street children's life world. They are emotionally evocative and provide insight into the children's hopes and dreams. On the one hand, the drawings are virtual mental maps of the surroundings in which the street children live. On the other hand, the highly personal nature of the material, often dealing with village and family life, show how drawing can be an effective instrument for coping with the past (Luig). The street is both the site of identity formation and the stigma children and youths in public spaces must deal with. By focussing on the drawings of two youths in particular, the distinctive and traumatic world of 'street children' comes into view. Children and youths are responsible subjects, with a considerable effect on society via adaptation, resistance or other innovative strategies of change. In this respect, they are creative social actors, actively constructing their life circumstances within society's framework (Luig and Seebode 19). Street drawings bring some of these strategies and processes to light.

Life World

Schütz modified Husserl's concept of the life world by adding his concept of 'everyday reality' (*Alltag*). The 'everyday world' (*Alltagswelt*) is the reality in which each human being thinks, feels, lives, acts and communicates. This world is given to each one of us and is accepted naturally and without questioning.

Through individual interaction with the material and social world, the life world is created and the individual horizon of experiences is expanded; this experience of the life world strongly influences the way human beings act (cf. Lave and Wenger). The life world is divided into the separate fields of being in which the individual becomes active, and individuals need a certain amount of knowledge and competency in order to function adequately in these surroundings; without it, disturbances occur which produce problems, such as anxiety. On the other hand, successful participation in one's fields of being produces feelings of individual security. Subjective feelings of identification and belonging can be obtained by adhering to the rules, norms and values of the particular field. In this case, the individual life world is embedded in societies' 'life world pattern' (*Lebensweltmuster*), which constitutes the frame for all individual patterns of thought and interpretation (Dachtler 74–75; Schubert 166–80; Grathoff; Schütz and Luckmann).

Definition and Deconstruction of the Concept 'Street Child'

The criteria to define the 'typical street child' are numerous. A street child spends the majority of the day on the street and in some cases the night as well. 'Street' refers here to all public and social spaces that are either accessible to street children or made accessible by them. Family ties are either entirely broken or tenuous, and, even if the children are still in touch with their families, the legal guardians are no longer the psychological parents. The street is the children's most important field of being, and it is there that they are mainly shaped. Most activities of everyday life such as working, playing, eating, sleeping or maintaining social relations occur here without the children having any kind of special protection or care (Dachtler 21–22). When the term 'street children' is used in the following, it includes adolescents, since many twenty-year olds still live on the street in a very similar way to the younger ones.

Only some of the children who spend time on the street are actually 'street children'. In academic literature a distinction is made between children who live on the street ('children of the street') and those who earn money on the street for themselves and/or their families ('children on the street') (Donald and Swart-Kruger 169). Richter defines street children, the 'children of the street', as children who 'have abandoned (or have been abandoned by) their families, schools and immediate communities, before they are sixteen years of age, and (have) drifted into a nomadic street life' (1). According to Glauser this definition is problematic in that children may alternate between a life on the street and temporary periods at relatives' and/or friends' places, or in welfare institutions or in prison. Therefore, it appears reasonable to assume that there is a continuum between the two groups, with the categorisation of any given individual to be determined by his or her circumstances (Aptekar and Abebe 480).

'Street child' itself is a problematic term because it hints at the traumatic aspects of such children's lives, such as their delinquency and the violence they encounter. It locates the streets as a place of illegal and criminal activity. This stresses the urgency in helping these children, for whom the streets are necessary to survival. The term suggests an exclusively negative sense of identity for the child without a family, home, or school to attend (cf. Schibotto; Liebel; Glauser). Schibotto emphasises the agency of these children and subjective capacities which enable urban survival. These children are essentially 'working children' (134) with lots of experience concerning the freedom of autonomy and inventing ways to overcome daily struggles. For the street children in question, their environment plays a crucial role in the development of identity and self-image. Through Luig and Seebode (19–20), we can call the street a *learning place*. These are places where children[2] and youths take responsibility for themselves and generate needed income through both formal and informal methods. This term underlines the meaning of learning as the acquisition of social capital; this especially serves children and youths who are not in legally protected situations with better chances for survival and education.

Drawings

Sengondo (twenty-two-year old) and Masumbuko (nineteen-year old)—these are pseudonyms and their real signatures have been removed from the drawings—are two youths who draw postcards which they try to sell to tourists. This is supported by a Christian aid project, and this faith is mirrored in the motifs chosen for the cards: Jesus in the manger and on the cross, complemented by indigenous, traditional village scenery and animals. Many motifs combine elements from the modern technical world, such as helicopters, military vehicles and radar antennas, with biblical content. To the eyes of tourists, the results are often absurd and disturbing collages which become a metaphor for the contradictory situation the street children live in (Figures 1 and 2).

I asked Sengondo and Masumbuko to illustrate their biographies and scenes of daily street life in Mwanza. In doing so, I did not further specify my request but instead let the boys themselves decide what they considered relevant. Both were paid for the drawings. After the drawings were completed, we talked about them. From over 100 drawings Sengondo and Masumbuko produced, this paper selects some examples of their work that offer insights to the inner world of street children. One of the village drawings in this paper was drawn by Masumbuko, and all the other drawings were drawn by Sengondo. Except for the drawing 'Street Kids', I have provided the titles for the drawings.

Sengondo has drawn many village drawings depicting a very happy, idealised way of life with everyone having enough to eat. These are ideals—wishes of how life ought to be (Figure 3).

Masumbuko, however, describes his village existence very differently. No ideals, instead a representation of great injustice; in Masumbuko's pictures men are exerting power over and violence on a boy. This drawing illustrates how a man

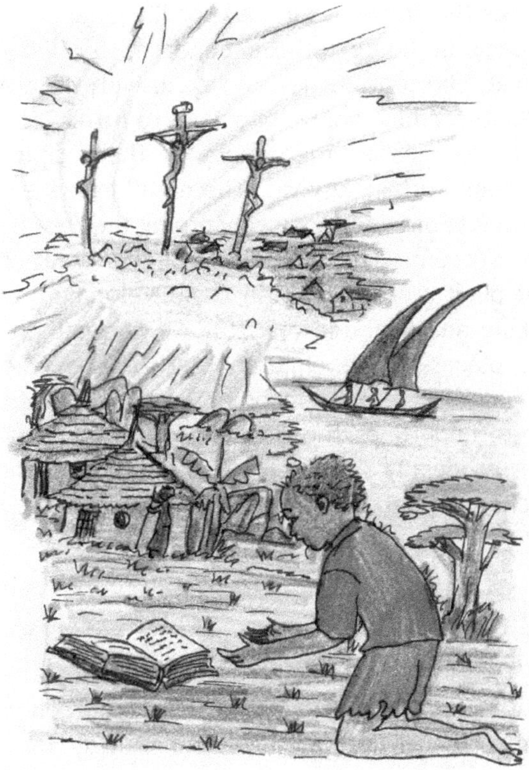

Figure 1 Jesus on the Cross.

chases a boy with the intent of beating him with a stick. Meanwhile someone is observing the scene from the door without intervening (Figure 4).

The picture 'Street Kids' gives an impression of the city of Mwanza. Here we are confronted with a situation at a bus station. It concisely represents the life world of street children. In contrast to the village scenes or depictions of children at play, this drawing does not depict rural influences; instead, we are presented with a busy urban setting with only asphalt, cars and buildings. At first, the viewer scans the group of children in the foreground. Then with closer observation certain other elements become apparent, with each person in their own state of poverty and neglect. Some wear tattered or simple clothes and others are barefoot. A striking consistency in Sengondo's work is the depiction of children as street dwellers. There seems to be no attention given to children with a relatively safe and stable existence (Figure 5).

In interviews I have been told by both male and female interviewees that most street girls were prostitutes. It was said to be the easiest way of earning money. Schibotto (134) points out that the term 'street girl' is used synonymously for *prostitute* in many languages.

Street boys perform other work to obtain money or food. Some work in the harbour, loading and unloading ships that mostly bear fish and fruit. Others collect pieces of wire to make fishing hooks to sell to the fishermen or go fishing

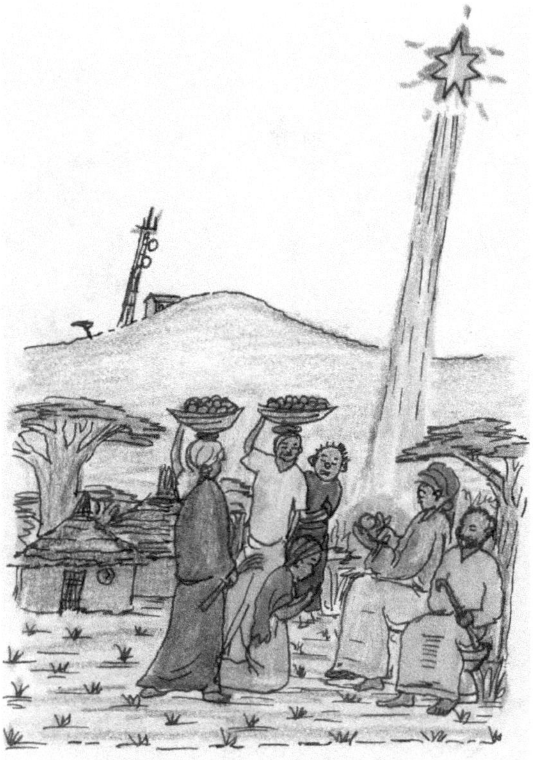

Figure 2 Radar antennas.

and either sell the catch or eat it themselves. Opportunities for work are also offered by the markets in the midst of the city: street boys help transport goods to and fro and do cleaning work; they sell eggs, milk, fruit, cigarettes, sweets or chewing gum; some also collect pieces of coal and aluminium rubbish to sell on; they work in restaurants and bars in town, performing menial tasks and receiving food as payment. It is impossible to walk through Mwanza without being approached by begging street children. Older children are particularly worse off, as they are rarely given anything. A fifteen-year old street boy explains:[3]

> He said at the beginning he was very young. And he could go, and on the way they could feel mercy and give him some money, one hundred or two hundred. He said, but now it's hard because he is going to growing up, so he cannot ask money, and they cannot give him because they see he is going to be old. (10th interview)

Another strategy of survival is theft: Sengondo's picture 'Harbour Theft' shows how a man is robbed by a boy and a girl pulling his money out of his pocket. The background shows two cranes, a ship and two cars. The theft as such seems small and unimportant. The victim seems wealthy, and that not only because of his tie. Interestingly, both children seem to be working hand in hand. These three figures appear to form a human chain, unloading the riches from the newly anchored

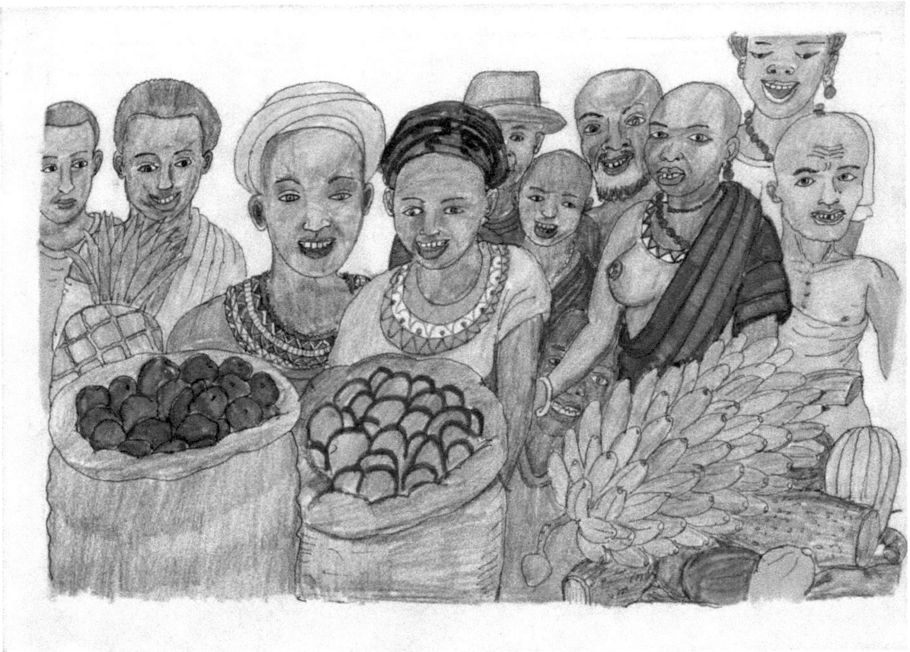

Figure 3 Harvest.

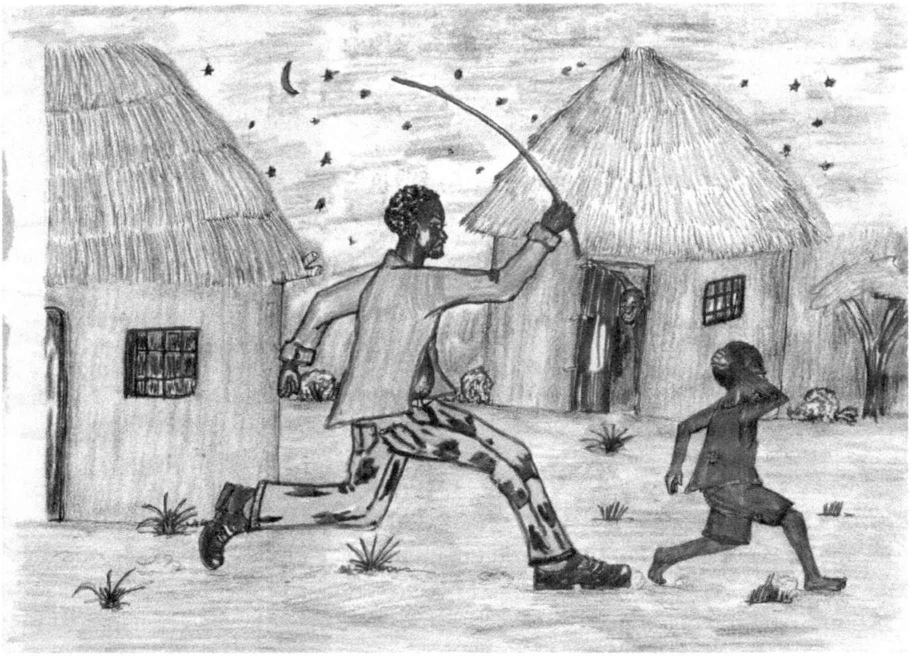

Figure 4 Chasing man.

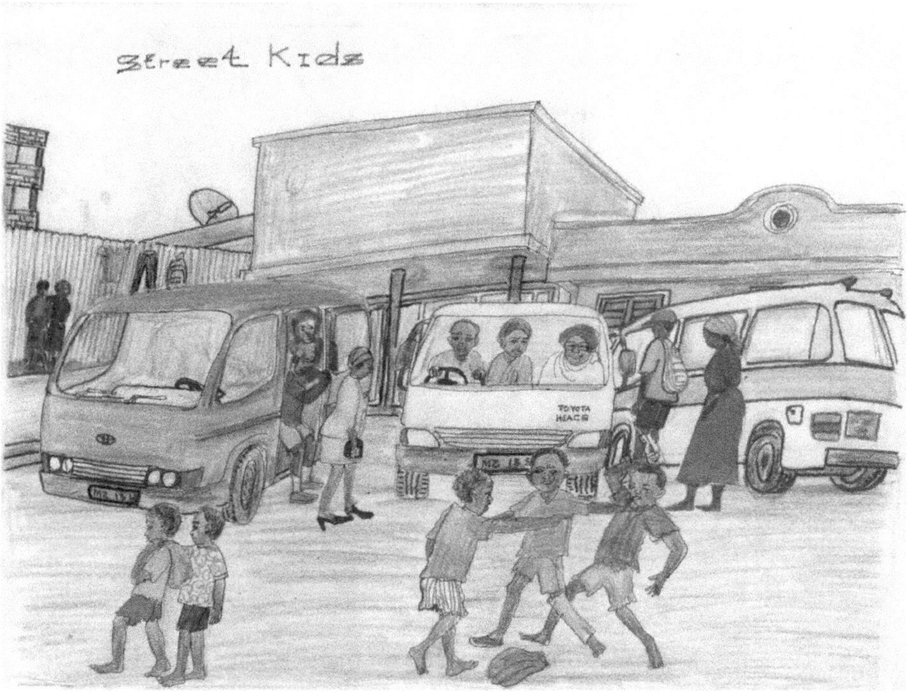

Figure 5 Street kids.

vessel, suggesting that street children too grasp the influences of globalisation and the economy (Figure 6).

In the work titled 'The Story of Maneno', two girls steal from an unsuspecting man's pocket. Interestingly, these street children are working together. While the girl in the red dress distracts the man, the other girl swiftly empties his back pocket. In the act of kneeling, she seems to be making a gesture of silence toward heaven, suggesting her consciousness of committing a Christian sin. Such a scene illustrates the main cause of societal prejudice directed at street children. But Sengondo eases the situation with an impression that is meant to be considered humorous (Figure 7).

In 'Glue-sniffers', five street boys are holding bottles of glue, while some on the left sniff them. This portrayal of social despair and desperation is reinforced by the background image of a car wreck under a tree. On the right side of the drawing, a boy is having an obvious dispute with someone who appears to be a businessman—he carries a briefcase and a mobile phone attached to his belt. The boy also holds a bottle of glue in his hand. But unlike his counterparts, he displays a level of resolution, attitude and presence of mind—sobering characteristics not often attributed to glue-sniffers. The overall impression of community between the glue-sniffers only emerges when the compositions are seen together. In the first view, we are left with no signs of solidarity beyond the joint activity of glue-sniffing. Each individual carries this out in their own self-determined way and there is no interaction between them. Yet there seems to be an invisible chain that links the boys on the left in their unspoken support of the

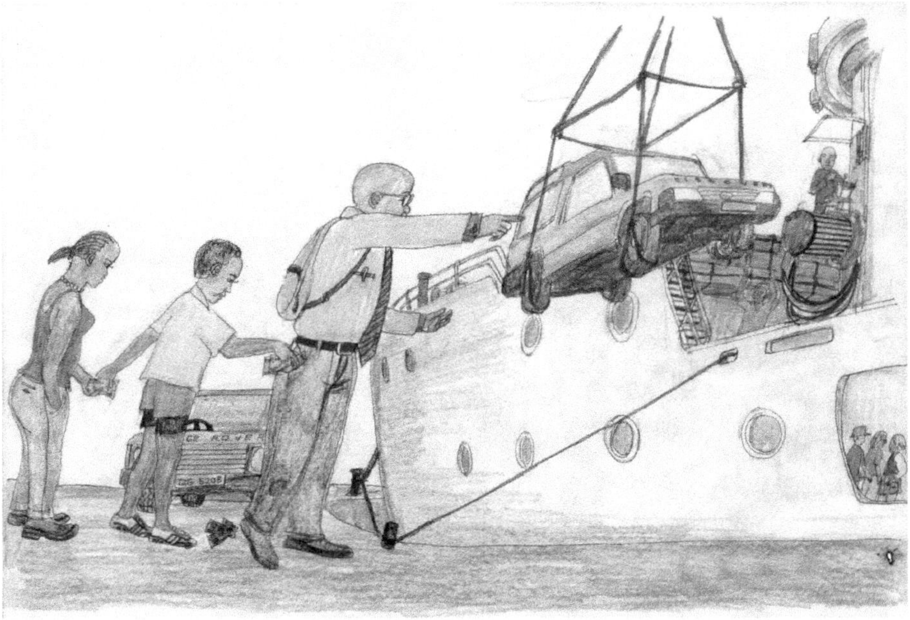

Figure 6 Harbour theft.

boy on the far right. The wrecked car keeps the figures optically together, which might also be seen as a connector of separate worlds, and representatives from these contrasting worlds now face each other: the businessman, who is socially integrated and might have driven the car when it still functioned, and the societal outsiders who stagnate like broken-down cars. For the viewer the drawing thus becomes a metaphor for the street children who are excluded from society, and for whom, just like car wrecks, there is no room in urban life (Figure 8).

In 'Police', we are shown a night time scene by the lake. A club-wielding policeman is carrying a crying boy by his shorts. In the distance, another policeman seems to hunt three additional street children. For Sengondo, the police uniform apparently holds a lot of significance since it is drawn in great detail. Even the emblems and digital watch on the policeman's wrist are clearly illustrated. It almost seems like the boy does not even want to fend off the policeman's violence, for in spite of being threatened by the club, he is still holding his cigarette in his hand instead of using it to defend himself (Figure 9).

The street children constitute a disturbance to the public sphere and as such are constantly confronted by state violence. When discussing the police, one must differentiate between the state police and private militias. The latter, which are called *sungusungu* in Kiswahili, are not always officially paid. Although I myself have been unable to observe any use of excessive violence by the police or the *sungusungu*, the interviews again and again show vehement and concurring reports of such violence. It is said that the police prefer to beat the joints of their

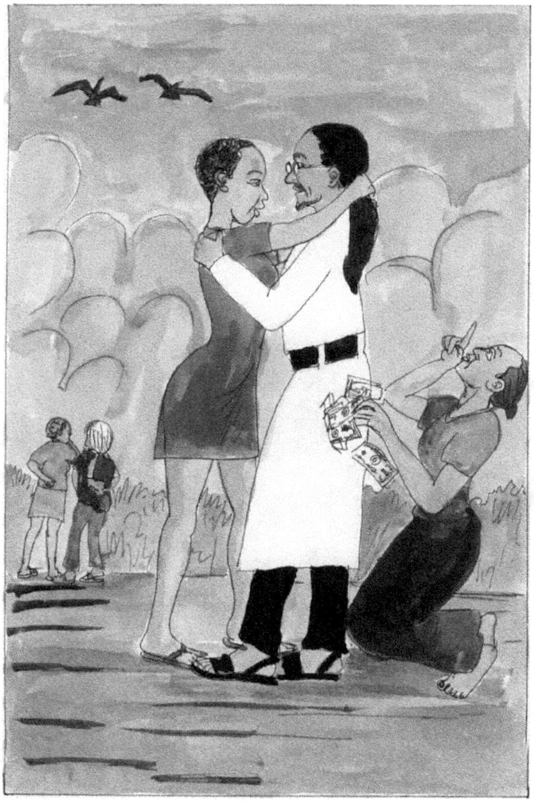

Figure 7 The story of Maneno.

victims, as no external bleeding occurs. A nineteen-year old male interviewee says:

> So the policemen come, always come to beat him, to disturb where you are sleeping. [. . .] The traditional police and police are altogether, and then they hit street children. If they want to meet you somewhere, they hit when you are sleeping under floor, they just hit you there. (ninth interview)

Regarding the traditional police there are also more differentiated statements which, however, do not change in their essential content.

> He says ah *sungusungu*, the traditional police, they fear the group of street children. He says they normally catch you when you are just yourself. (eleventh interview, twenty-year old male)

Girls are subjected to both physical and sexual abuse.

> She says when you have no money to policemen, they just ask you to sex, they make sexual abuse, and when you are not receiving, accepting, they fight you. (sixteenth interview, seventeen-year old female)

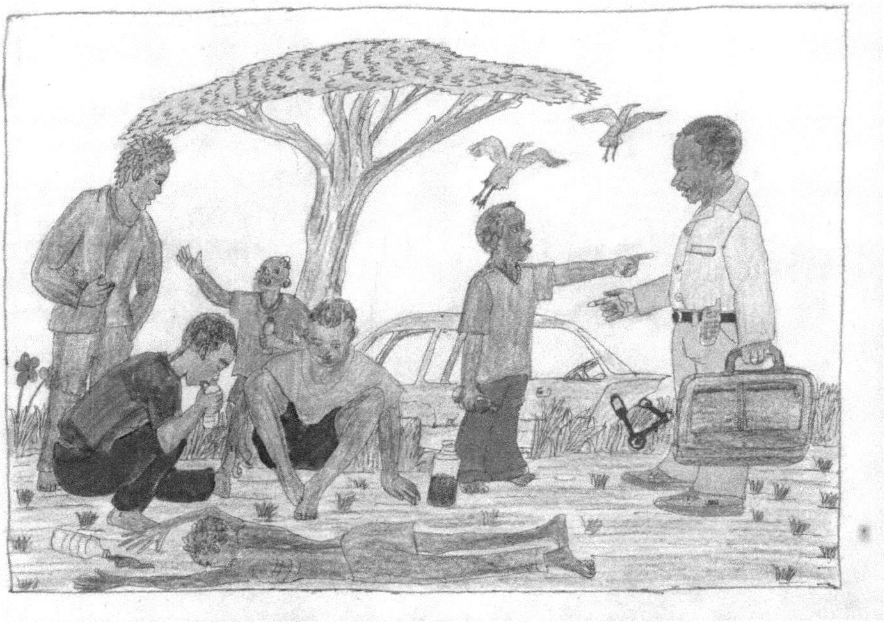

Figure 8 Glue sniffers.

An eighteen-year old female interviewee describes the situation as follows:

> She says there are problems of policemen catching you as a girl and be sending you somewhere to do sexual abuse. And then there are many, not one because policemen—I don't know why—they just come many. And then they keep you on secret, and they do some things, such kind of things. And then after this ah because they have done once, she says, they took me there, and they have done so many things, something like that. (twentieth interview)

The work called 'Terminator' is a self-generated poster for the movie 'Terminator 2' in which some parts bear resemblance to the official version. Like the original poster, Sengondo's rendition is separated into two halves—the inner and outer. On the right side, Sengondo shows the intact, carnal half of the face of the protagonist. In addition, he is shown on his motorcycle. The left reveals the peculiar machine identity that lies beneath the human-like facade of the Terminator. Here the machine body rises from the flames to form a duality with its carnal embodiment—the motorcyclist hero. The flames have left a path of destruction and only ghastly human skulls remain.

The Terminator is a classic hero. He arrives in our time as a robot from the future to rescue a boy who will eventually save mankind. This 'revolution in the future' will threaten the existence of humanity as they face a dangerous new robot species. The Terminator's technical inferiority to this improved generation of robots brings him closer to the side of human beings. Although he remains a machine, he acts with a 'good heart'. Consequently, the hero is faced with a

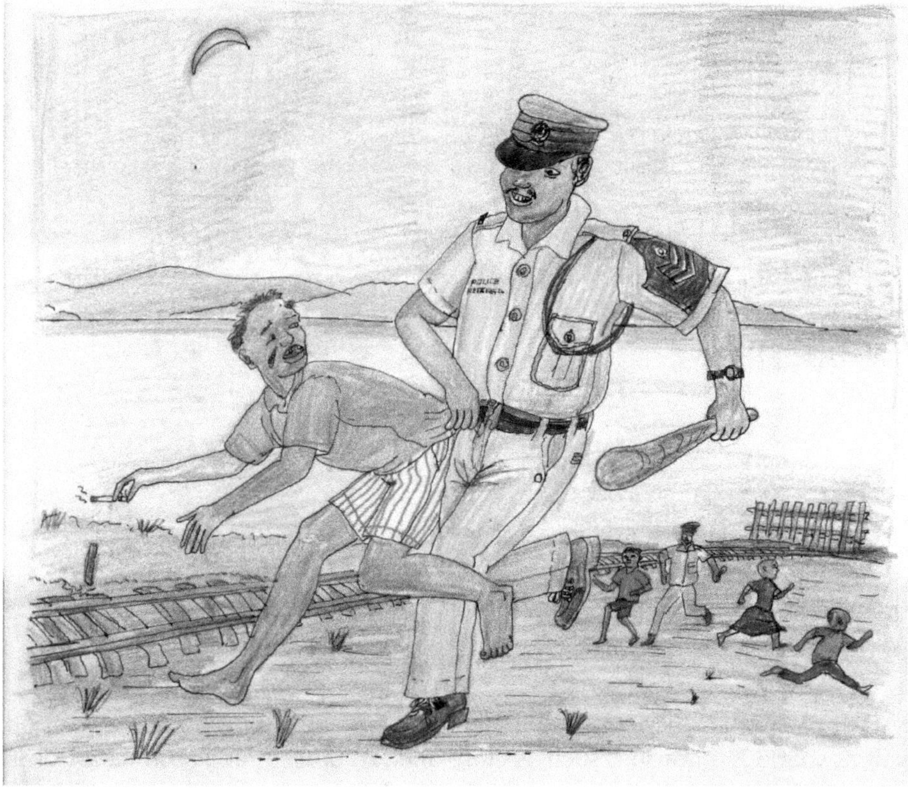

Figure 9 Police.

tragic decision; self-sacrifice for the rescue of mankind. Does he belong to the laws of his programming as a machine, or his 'good heart'? For the Terminator, only his own morality is relevant. With the title 'Judgement Day', the strong Christian reference is obvious (Figure 10).

Street Children and Urban Space

The life world of the street children is inseparable from the urban environment in which they live. When, in the course of the processes of globalisation, children and youths migrate to the cities, the spatial organisation of their social relationships changes. These processes of change are also reflected in the differences between the village and city drawings. Social relationships always have a spatial form and a spatial content (Massey 168–69). The city brings with it a different moral order, in which the position and self-awareness of the street children is defined anew by the attitudes and standards of other individuals and groups. The meaning of their newly prescribed social status is social distance. And social distance stands in close relation to spatial distance, as physical distance is also an index for social distance (Park 17–18). As the fundamental

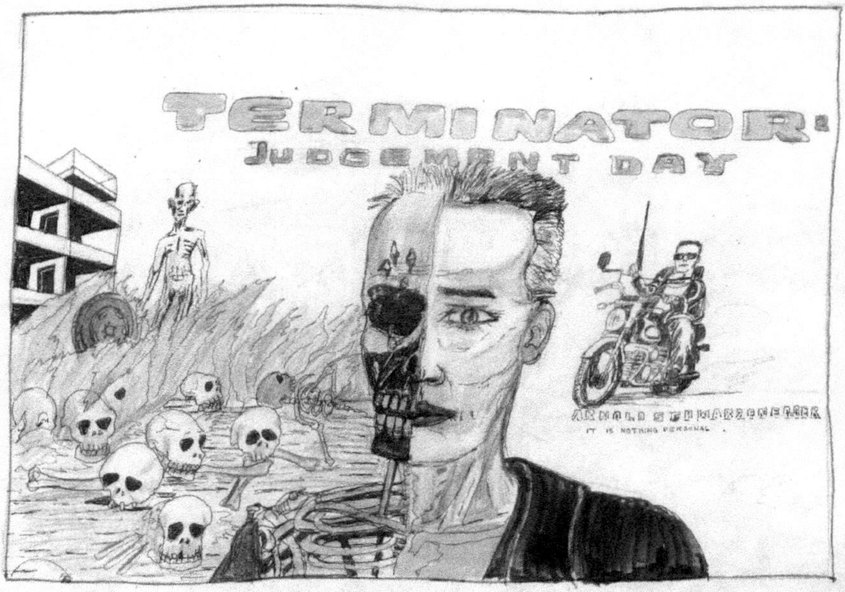

Figure 10 Terminator.

system of spatial divisions like subject and object, inclusion and exclusion, as well as spatial separations such as close and far, present and absent, cultural and natural, space determines social points of reference for perception which in turn generates the hegemonic system of ideology and practice. The spatial preconditions constitute cultural perceptions and prejudices, and establish performative codes which link social practices and ways of social interaction to their respective milieu. In this respect, spatial concepts manifest themselves in societal discourses. They play an important role in justifying and legitimising everyday decisions and actions (cf. Lakoff and Johnson). The spatial separations are also constitutive for social separations between groups (Shields 46–47). In his drawings 'Glue-Sniffers' and 'Police', Sengondo depicts these social separations between groups very clearly. The street children's urban living environment is not ontologically defined at the outset, but receives its meaning as social space when its residents discursively and physically define it in their everyday lives (De Certeau). When children have to live on the streets they first of all have to learn about how such a context operates. If they achieve this they can then start to manipulate it with practice.

The street children, as social actors, create their own realities and meanings within public space. However, the street children occupy spaces which were not intended for them, and they thus threaten the social order. The children who come to Mwanza initially stand on a threshold as they turn into street children; in this transitional space the process of identity formation takes place.

In the interviews and in songs and drawings, they represent themselves as 'street children' and separate from society. Survival strategies and everyday life reveal strong similarities amongst all the children. Other members of society generally distance themselves from them and associate them with theft in particular and menace more generally. In return, the street children feel they do not belong to society, that they are different. Street children are very strongly socialised at a young age by the others: new arrivals meet with hardened social structures and behavioural patterns which are assimilated. In the transitional space of the street, the children come together through their participation in street life, the shared experiences, and the resulting trust, and they form social networks, within which they receive social support. The representation of the street children's perspective in their drawings and other media allows other people (including those in the international community) to apparently enter their world whilst giving them attention, understanding and sympathy. But simultaneously, social norms are sustained, and borders between the street children and 'normality' are evident. Street children are in this sense stigmatised, marginalised and discriminated against; many studies of street children in different societies show that the biggest fear amongst the children is the enmity of the public and the police (Aptekar and Abebe 477), and that they are subjected to manifold forms of abuse.

Conclusion

In 2004, three years on from my interviews, my translator from 2001 attempted to re-question my interview partners. Of the original twenty-two interview partners, fourteen could no longer be found. Six boys had emigrated to another city, one had found a job, one was in prison, and another one was in the new centre of an aid project. Of the unavailable girls, one had died of AIDS, two continued to live on the street in Mwanza, and another two had gone to Dar es Salaam. The re-interviewed youths gave differing statements on the developments over the previous three years. For some the situation had greatly improved. Thus, one young man and one young woman worked with an aid project. Two girls and four boys continued to live on the street, and one boy was in prison.

The renewed questioning confirms that street children and youths are social actors whose biographies can take relatively different courses. Street children are active contributors who can reshape their position in the social arena (i.e. by creating networks and ultimately supporting themselves). To invoke Bourdieu, they can earn social capital which orientates them with the society at large and gives them control over their lives in a more constructive way. Instead of emphasising the vulnerability and victimisation of street children (as it is often done in the media and the advertising of aid organisations), examining their drawings and other self representations suggests the street children's abilities to deal with the difficulties of daily life. In their art we see autobiographical representations that incorporate the signs and symbols of their life world, and distinctive intersubjective and cross cultural formations that shape the life world of Mwanza's children and youths of the streets (Wiencke).

Notes

[1] This article is a summarised and further revised version of material that has previously been published in a book. I am especially grateful to my German publisher IKO-Verlag für Interkulturelle Kommunikation (Frankfurt am Main, London) for giving permission to use parts of my book: *Straßenkinder in Tansania. Ihre Lebenswelt in der Stadt Mwanza* (*Street Children in Tanzania. Their Life World in the City of Mwanza*), 2007. Additionally, I would like to thank Katrin Hennicke for the translation.

[2] Luig and Seebode relate the concept to youths only.

[3] I worked with a translator who was a street boy.

References

Aptekar, Lewis, and Behailu Abebe. 'Conflict in the Neighbourhood. Street and Working Children in the Public Space.' *The International Journal of Children's Rights* 5.4 (1997): 477–90.

Bourdieu, Pierre. 'Ökonomisches Kapital, kulturelles Kapital, soziales Kapital.' *Soziale Ungleichheiten* ['Economic Capital, Cultural Capital, Social Capital.' *Social Inequalities*]. Ed. Reinhard Kreckel. Göttingen, Ger.: Nomos, 1983. 183–98.

Dachtler, Armin. *Die Straßenkinder in Tansania. Darstellung ihrer Lebenswelt am Beispiel der Stadt Bukoba* [*Street Children in Tanzania. Depictions of Their Life World Using the Example of the City of Bukoba*]. Frankfurt am Main, Ger.: IKO, 1999.

De Certeau, Michel. *The Practice of Everyday Life*. Berkeley,CA, Los Angeles, CA: U of California P, 1988.

Donald, David, and Jill Swart-Kruger. 'The South African Street Child: Developmental Implications.' *South African Journal of Psychology* 24.4 (1994): 169–74.

Geertz, Clifford. *Dichte Beschreibung. Beiträge zum Verstehen kultureller Systeme* [*Thick Description: Toward an Interpretive Theory of Culture*]. 6th ed. Frankfurt am Main, Ger.: Suhrkamp, 1999.

Glauser, Benno. 'Street Children: Deconstructing a Construct.' *Constructing and Reconstructing Childhood: Contemporary Issues in the Sociological Study of Childhood*. 2nd ed. Eds. Allison James, and Alan Prout. London, Gt. Brit.: Falmer Press, 1997. 145–64.

Grathoff, Richard. *Milieu und Lebenswelt. Einführung in die phänomenologische Soziologie und die sozial-phänomenologische Forschung* [*Milieu and Life World. An Introduction to Phenomenological Sociology and Social Phenomenological Research*]. Frankfurt am Main, Ger.: Suhrkamp, 1995.

Husserl, Edmund. 'Das Problem der Lebenswelt.' *Edmund Husserl. Phänomenologie der Lebenswelt. Ausgewählte Texte II* [*'The Problem of the Life World.' Edmund Husserl. Phenomenology of the Life World. Selected Texts II*]. Ed. Klaus Held. Stuttgart, Ger.: Reclam, 2002. 220–92.

Lakoff, George, and Mark Johnson. *Metaphors We Live by*. Chicago: U of Chicago P, 2003.

Lave, Jean, and Etienne Wenger. *Situated Learning. Legitimate Peripheral Participation*. Cambridge: Cambridge UP, 1991.

Liebel, Manfred. 'Vorwort.' *Unsichtbare Kindheit. Kinder in der informellen Ökonomie ['Preface.' Invisible Childhood. Children within the Informal Economy]*. Ed. Giangi Schibotto. Frankfurt am Main, Ger.: IKO, 1993. 10–14.

Luig, Ute. 'Vorwort.' Straßenkinder in Tansania. Ihre Lebenswelt in der Stadt Mwanza ['Preface.' Street Children in Tanzania. Their Life World in the City of Mwanza]. Ed. Markus Wiencke. Frankfurt am Main, Ger., London, Gt. Brit.: IKO, 2007. 7–8.

Luig, Ute, and Jochen Seebode. 'Einleitung. Ethnologie der Jugend: Soziale Praxis, moralische Diskurse und inszenierte Körperlichkeit.' *Ethnologie der Jugend. Soziale Praxis, moralische Diskurse und inszenierte Körperlichkeit* ['Introduction. Anthropology of Youth: Social Practices, Moral Discourses and Representation of the Body'. *Anthropology of Youth: Social Practices, Moral Discourses and Representation of the Body*]. Eds. Ute Luig, and Jochen Seebode. Münster, Ger.: LIT, 2003. 9–40.

Massey, 1994. Massey, Doreen. 'A Place Called Home.' *Space, Place and Gender.* Ed. Doreen Massey. Cambridge, MA: Polity Press, 1994. 157–73.

Matt, Eduard. 'Darstellung qualitativer Forschung.' *Qualitative Forschung – ein Handbuch* ['Presentation of Qualified Research.' *Qualitative Research – a Manual*]. 2nd ed. Eds. Uwe Flick, Ernst von Kardorff, and Ines Steinke. Reinbek, Ger.: Rowohlt, 2003. 578–87.

Mayring, Philipp. 'Qualitative Inhaltsanalyse.' *Qualitative Forschung – ein Handbuch* ['Qualitative Content Analysis.' *Qualitative Research – a Manual*]. 2nd ed. Eds. Uwe Flick, Ernst von Kardorff, and Ines Steinke. Reinbek, Ger.: Rowohlt, 2003. 468–75.

Park, Robert E. 'The Urban Community as a Spatial Pattern and a Moral Order.' *The Urban Community.* Ed. Ernest W. Burgess. Chicago: Chicago UP, 1926. 3–18.

Richter, Linda M. 'Street Children: the Nature and Scope of the Problem in Southern Africa.' *The Child Care Worker* 6 (1988): 11–14.

Schibotto, Giangi. *Unsichtbare Kindheit. Kinder in der informellen Ökonomie [Invisible Childhood. Children within the Informal Economy]*. Frankfurt am Main, Ger.: IKO, 1993.

Schubert, Franz-Christian. 'Lebensweltorientierte Sozialarbeit – Grundpostulate, Selbstverständnis und Handlungsperspektiven.' *Professionelle Identitäten in der Sozialarbeit/ Sozialpädagogik: Anstöße, Herausforderungen und Rahmenbedingungen im Prozess der Entwicklung eines beruflichen Selbstverständnisses ['Life-world-oriented Social Work. Basic Assumptions, Self-conception and Perspectives of Action.' Professional Identities within Social Work/Social Pedagogy: Ideas, Challenges and Basic Conditions in the Process of Developing a Professional Self-conception]*. Ed. Wilhelm Klüsche. Mönchengladbach, Ger.: Fachhochschule Niederrhein [University of Applied Science of Niederrhein], Fachbereich Sozialwesen [Social Studies Department], 1994. 165–211.

Schütz, Alfred. *Der sinnhafte Aufbau der sozialen Welt. Eine Einleitung in die verstehende Soziologie [The Phenomenology of the Social World. An Introduction to Interpretative Sociology]*. Frankfurt am Main, Ger.: Suhrkamp, 1974

Schütz, Alfred, and Thomas Luckmann. *Strukturen der Lebenswelt [Structures of the Life World]*. Vols. 1 and 2. Frankfurt am Main, Ger.: Suhrkamp, 1979.

Shields, Rob. 'Alternative geographies of modernity.' *Places on the Margin: Alternative Geographies of Modernity.* Ed. Rob Shields. London, Gt. Brit., New York: Routledge, 1991. 29–70

Spradley, James P. *The Ethnographic Interview.* New York: Holt, Rinehart and Winston, 1979.

Spradley, James P. *Participant Observation.* New York: Holt, Rinehart and Winston, 1980.

Wiencke, Markus. *Straßenkinder in Tansania. Ihre Lebenswelt in der Stadt Mwanza [Street Children in Tanzania. Their Life World in the City of Mwanza]*. Frankfurt am Main, Ger., London, Gt. Brit.: IKO, 2007.

Witzel, Andreas. 'Das problemzentrierte Interview.' *Qualitative Sozialforschung in der Psychologie* ['The Problem-centred Interview.' *Qualitative Social Research in Psychology*]. 2nd ed. Ed. Gerd Jüttemann. Weinheim, Ger.: Beltz, 1989. 227–55.

Wolff, Stephan. 'Wege ins Feld und ihre Varianten.' *Qualitative Forschung – ein Handbuch* ['Paths into the Field and their Variants.' *Qualitative Research – a Manual*]. 2nd ed. Eds. Uwe Flick, Ernst von Kardorff, and Ines Steinke. Reinbek, Ger.: Rowohlt, 2003. 475–85.

Testimonio and Telling Women's Narratives of Genocide, Torture and Political Imprisonment in Post-Suharto Indonesia

Annie Pohlman

> Then, in 1965, then the troubles and upheaval came, the political strife came. And I was washed away by it, destroyed by it. (Ibu Eny)[1]

In the aftermath of a military coup in Jakarta on the night of 30 September 1965, an estimated half a million people were murdered and a further one and a half million imprisoned for their alleged involvement.[2] The regime which seized power in the months following the coup and which perpetrated the massacres, General Suharto's New Order, remained in power until 1998. In the years since the fall of the regime, efforts have been made to initiate a Truth and Reconciliation Commission in Indonesia which would investigate human rights abuses perpetrated under the New Order, including the massacre and mass political detention of 'coup sympathisers'. To date, however, any official investigation into human rights abuses under the New Order has failed to take place.

In the absence of official processes, the non-legal arenas in which survivors' stories are told and the political and cultural landscapes of post-Suharto Indonesia which allow or prohibit their telling are vitally important. The narratives of women survivors in particular have been occluded and silenced, and the work of collecting, documenting and analysing their stories is now urgent. *Testimonio* is the political and analytical framework I will draw upon here. Those aspects of *testimonio* which demand a response from the reader, underline the inescapable presence of multiple voices within the narratives, and draw attention to the situation of urgency and trauma from which these testimonies arise are essential in the continuing negotiations over who can speak, about what, and with what result in post-Suharto Inconesia. Specific discursive strategies found within the narratives highlight some of the issues which permit or proscribe the articulation of certain stories. Most particularly, the context of narration when relating experiences of sexual violence perpetrated against women during the killings and political detention reveals certain strategies of how women discursively negotiate describing, or not describing, these assaults.

Histories of 1965

During its long-lasting authoritarian, militarist reign, the New Order created, adapted and policed its narrative of the 1965 coup and the events which followed to shape its official version of history. According to this narrative, the Indonesian Communist Party had orchestrated the failed coup d'état. The Indonesian military, led by General Suharto, responded to the threat posed by Communism and, in defence of the nation, eradicated those responsible for the coup in order to save Indonesia. Under the New Order, those murdered or detained were branded ruthless 'betrayers' of the nation. The propaganda campaign following the coup effectively discredited communist ideology and cultivated the association of communism with perversion, immorality and betrayal.[3] Throughout the New Order, the regime continually evoked the spectre of 'latent communism' to justify and maintain its authoritarian rule. Essentially, because the regime claimed that it had 'saved' the nation from the communist aborted coup (and because they were ever vigilant of such a threat arising again), this warranted its long-lasting authoritarian rule. As Ariel Heryanto explains, this 'master narrative secured the regime's legitimacy, and served an indispensable function in the protracted political "stability and order"' of the New Order (153).

Other histories of 1965 and the New Order's legacy emerge covertly:

> Near my old house there was a betel palm tree, and they'd slaughter [people] there near the mountain top. They'd be pulled along by their feet, at the mountain near my old home, suspended by their feet, by their hands. This happened when I was already in prison, but my daughter told me about it. They'd

> put the wooden stick in here (she mimes a long stick being placed between her legs and hands), like they were carrying a pig. After they cut [the victim's throat], blood would spill out everywhere. They'd all come down together, [calling], 'We've got one! We've got a pig!' (Ibu Eny)

Ibu Eny currently lives on the outskirts of a small village in Sumatra. As with many who were members of organisations associated with the Indonesian Communist Party, when the coup occurred in Jakarta in October 1965, once the military's propaganda spread blaming the coup on the Communists, she followed her organisation's orders to flee the cities. She, her husband and a number of others who were also organisation members, attempted to hide in the villages and forests in West Sumatra. They were apprehended by the mob; her husband and the others were killed and she was left alive and taken for questioning.

Although she survived the killings, Ibu Eny became one of the estimated one-and-a-half million political prisoners or *tapols* (an abbreviation of *tahanan politik*) detained on a blanket charge of 'direct or indirect involvement in the 30 September Coup' (Tapol 1). Those imprisoned were most often subjected to interrogation, torture, starvation and forced labour in overcrowded and substandard prisons and detention centres (Flanagan and Southwood 3). The length of time individual *tapols* spent in prison varied; some were released after a few months while other, more 'serious Communists' were detained for more than ten years. One of the women who took part in this project, Ibu Lia, spent twenty-two years in prison. Ibu Eny was released after thirteen years in detention, never once having seen the inside of a courtroom.

Many of those who gave their testimonies as part my project expressed anger and bitterness at the lack of any legal processing during their detention; the vast majority of *tapols* were never charged or put on trial for the crimes for which they were held and for which many of their friends, family members or associates were murdered. This resentment for having been so arbitrarily detained was expressed by many former political prisoners during interviews. One man who had been imprisoned in one of the notoriously harsh prison camps on Buru Island echoed these responses: '[We] did nothing! [...] If we had been guilty, fine then, I would have been prepared to accept it. Take us to court, in front of the court, try [us]. But there was nothing! No [evidence] at all!'[4] Forty years on, the lack of any official investigation and redress of the crimes committed against them, such as would be carried out by a Truth and Reconciliation Commission, angers many. In 2005, twelve former political prisoners launched a class action suing former Presidents Suharto, Yusuf Habibie, Abdurrahman Wahid and Megawati Sukarnoputri as well as current President Susilo Bambang Yudhoyono for failing to restore their civil rights and the rights of millions of others accused of being communists (Kearney 21). When I raised this case during some interviews, although most believed that the attempt would fail, it was seen as a chance for survivors to testify about their experiences.[5] As one woman asserted, 'I never once saw the inside of a courtroom even though I was in prison for many years [...] I want my chance to stand before a court and say what happened'.[6]

Outside political and legal circles, however, alternative narratives to the New Order's version of history circulate. As Ann Laura Stoler noted in relation to the early years after the fall of Suharto, with the end of the New Order came an unprecedented 'explosion of interest' in discussing the Indonesian past and, in particular, the events following the 1965 coup (642). Prior to 1998, publications relating to 1965 which portrayed events differently from the regime were banned (Zurbuchen 571). Since 1998, numerous memoirs, collections of memoirs and accounts, and scholarly works about and by former political prisoners have been published and are widely available in Indonesia.[7]

Kay Schaffer and Sidonie Smith's work on the relationship between human rights' movements and life narratives is useful to consider this 'explosion of interest' in the events of 1965 in Indonesia. They draw attention to 'the importance of storytelling in bringing the specificities of local conditions of abuse ... to the attention of a global community' (20). One way that these narratives do so is by attaining what Gillian Whitlock refers to as a 'discursive threshold' (144). By examining emergent life narratives by black women in South Africa and Australia, Whitlock shows that it is not only necessary to analyse the narratives themselves but also essential to interrogate '[w]hat conditions created the enunciative space that these [testimonies] occupy' (144). Within post-Suharto Indonesia, where memoirs and accounts of 1965 are gaining increasing political and cultural distribution but where official processes have yet to begin, the collection and circulation of narratives may serve another function. As Schaffer and Smith have found, these women's narratives may help to 'generate climates that enable the reception and recognition of new stories' (4). In other words, when stories about events in the Indonesian past are published and circulated, this may, in turn, encourage others who survived these events (and other human rights abuses perpetrated by the New Order) to speak also.

Specific characteristics of *testimonio* offer a way for the narratives of women survivors of the 1965–66 killings and political imprisonment to achieve greater circulation both in and outside Indonesia. Yvonne Unnold asserts that there are three characteristics of *testimonios*; first, they emerge 'in a sociopolitical situation of urgency'; second, they 'are driven by the commitment to bear witness'; and lastly, they 'seek to transform a sociopolitical consciousness' (13). In response to more than forty years of political, social and economic repression, the survivors whose stories are emerging spoke their truths about their pasts in order to refute New Order discourses of history. In essence, the very existence of these testimonies, their *raison d'être*, originates from and constitutes a challenge to an opposing, official history.

Testimonio and Political Purpose

> [After my husband and the others were killed] then they took me to the police station. At the station I was 'processed' every day, every morning. In the mornings, the police would call us all for our [roll call], so I'd come out. I'd be

> processed again, I didn't want to answer their questions, so they'd hit me, beat me here, beat me here, hit me until my head swelled up ... Everyone was beaten! [...] Women, men, girls, all of us, people would be able to recognise us before we went in to be interrogated, but they wouldn't afterwards. There would be screams and crying from the beatings [...] We were tortured in many different ways. We were women, but they still beat us. They would beat us with long rubber rods, yelling, 'Confess!' If you didn't confess, you were beaten, but no-one confessed. But because we were hurt so badly, in the end, well, well, it was just ... it happened. (Ibu Eny)

One of the most important and distinctive features of *testimonio* is that the narratives are told in order to elicit a response in the reader/listener. As John Beverley's definition suggests, 'The situation of narration in *testimonio* [involves] an urgency to communicate' ('The Margin' 12–13). In the case of the testimonies by the survivors of 1965, the goal is to inform people about and involve them in the struggle by survivors in Indonesia to have the human rights' abuses perpetrated by the New Order regime acknowledged and redressed.

In order for these processes to take place, however, *testimonio*'s goals of informing readers about situations of urgency and involving them in these struggles must be achieved. The famous *testimonio*, *I, Rigoberta Menchu—An Indian Woman in Guatemala*, illustrates the potential power of the genre. Prior to the publication of Menchu's account in 1983, the massacres of Mayan people during the Guatemalan army's 'scorched earth' campaign in the early 1980s had gone largely unnoticed internationally. Despite the controversies which surround Menchu, particularly after the publication of David Stoll's *Rigoberta Menchu and the Story of All Poor Guatemalans*, her book is important for the discussion of the political aims of *testimonio* as, more than any other, it brought international attention and condemnation of the treatment of the Maya in Guatemala (Sanford 51).

Menchu's account suggests how *testimonio* aims to inform and involve the reader. It does so partly because, during the recording of the *testimonio*, the narrator is addressing the interlocutor who, as was the case during my own interviews with women survivors, will listen, ask questions and occasionally redirect the conversation. As Doris Sommer shows, however, this speaking with another person shifts, 'by extension, [to] each reader [who] is addressed by the narrator's immediate appeal to "you" ... When the narrator talks about her*self* to *you*, she implies both the existing relationship to other representative selves in the community and potential relationship that extend her community through the text' (118). While this is by no means a straightforward process, *testimonio* demands that the reader move from the subject positions of voyeur or tourist, to a position whereby s/he is required to *do something*. As Beverley explains: 'we are placed under an obligation to respond; we may act or not on that obligation, we may resent or welcome it, but we cannot ignore it' (*Testimonio* 1).

Multiple Subjects, Multiple Subjectivities

Georg Yudice's definition of *testimonio* highlights the narrator as 'an agent (rather than a representative) of a collective memory and identity' (17). This is another defining and controversial characteristic of *testimonio* as it complicates the issues of voice, subjectivity and representation, yet it is also an inexorable characteristic of the narratives of women survivors during the course of this project. The multiple subjects/subjectivities present within the testimonies also problematise other fundamental issues of *testimonio*, such as truth, history and authority. This was highlighted when Stoll's book challenged the veracity of Menchu's *testimonio*, claiming that it could not 'be the eyewitness account it purports to be' because some of the events she described were 'experiences she never had herself' (xii). As Leigh Gilmore explains:

> [W]hen the issue is narrowed to the legalistic question, 'Did she lie?,' almost none of the complexity of representing the self in the context of representing trauma can be retained ... her testimony tests a crucial limit ... and not just the one understood as the boundary between truth and lies, but, rather, the limit of representativeness, with its compulsory inflation of the self to stand for others, the particular way it operates both to expand and to constrict testimonial speech, and the way it makes it hard to clarify without falsifying what is strictly and unambiguously 'my' experience when 'our' experience is also at stake. (*Limits* 5)

Beverley explains that *testimonio* is less concerned with the life of the protagonist/narrator than 'with the problematic collective social situation that the narrator lives with or alongside others' ('The Margin' 15). The 'I' stands for many, not as a singular story but as the story of many in a situation of urgency. As L. P. Rice-Sayre writes in relation to Menchu's *testimonio*, 'It is not Menchu's uniqueness that makes her life story worth telling; rather, her life story is important because it repeats the experience of so many others' (52). In particular, for the purposes of this project, I investigate 'multiple *testimonios*', or, as Beverley describes them, 'polyphonic' *testimonios*, a 'formal variation on the classic ... singular *testimonio* ... made up of accounts by different participants in the same event' ('The Margin' 16). This type of testimonial writing is much closer to my attempt to present and analyse women survivors' testimonies of their experiences under the New Order in Indonesia. While straying far from a more 'prototypical'[8] model of *testimonio*, such as *I, Rigoberta Menchu*, by presenting the testimonies of a larger number of women who experienced similar events under the New Order, I understand each individual to be a spokesperson of a larger population of survivors of the mass killings and political imprisonment.

Trauma and Multiple Subjects

> Those of us with husbands who didn't come back meant that they were murdered, that's for certain. If they didn't come back, it meant that they couldn't come back. When we were released from jail, when we got home, if someone wasn't there, be it your child, your husband, your wife, your family, it meant that they were dead, that was it. (Ibu Eny)

When those who were imprisoned, such as Ibu Eny who spent thirteen years in jail, were finally released, they often returned home to find members of their families missing or frightened to be associated with them due to the stigma of political imprisonment. The former prisoners also returned home to face restrictions on freedoms of movement, speech, political participation and other rights. These restrictions were further expanded during the 1980s with the enforcement of such policies as the 'Clean Self, Clean Environment' policy which curtailed not only the rights of former political prisoners, but also those of their families. In essence, the Institute for National Defence recommended that Indonesian citizens be 'clean' and 'clean in their surroundings', the latter a reference to a person's relationships with former political prisoners. As a result of the government's stance on this issue, 'certificates of non-involvement in the 30 September Movement/Indonesian Communist Party' were required of any person seeking employment in government services, the military and some businesses, as well as for admission to school or university, or of anyone wishing to move to a new district (van der Kroef 643). Thus, the individual women who gave their testimonies as part of this project often emphasised the ever-expanding sphere of influence of this collective trauma; a trauma which they experienced as individuals, as inmates within prison camps which held hundreds if not thousands, and as members within families who, by association, also suffered the Suharto government's vigilant repression of 'latent communism'.

The individual's ability to represent the trauma experienced by many has also been dealt with by a number of Holocaust survivors and scholars. Discussing the concentration camps of Nazi-occupied Europe, Terrence Des Pres draws attention to the conditions of these camps where the identities of individuals were erased, where 'men and women were reduced to a single human mass' (37). When the survivors of the camps began to speak about their experiences, they would often speak using the first person plural; 'Almost all survivors say "we" rather than "I" when describing their camp experiences' (Des Pres 29). Kathryn Robson also examines Holocaust survivors' attempts to represent trauma and draws our attention to Charlotte Delbo's trilogy, *Auschwitz et Après*, in which she bears witness not only to her own experiences but also to those of her fellow inmates in Auschwitz-Birkenau and Ravensbrück as well as to the survivors' lives after returning to France (157). The third part of the trilogy, *Mesure de Nos Jours*, appears to be a collection of narratives by different people who had been in the camps—both those who survived as well as those who did not. Each of the narratives, all written by Delbo, 'brings with it a testimonial obligation: to bear witness to the trauma suffered by a silenced collective, to speak for those who cannot' (Robson 158). Des Pres and Delbo both illustrate how '[c]ollective trauma appears to render individual testimony problematic, as the individual's experience of mass trauma is tightly interwoven with that of the collective' (Robson 158). For Des Pres, 'Survival is a collective act, and so is bearing witness' (38). As can be seen in Delbo's trilogy, whether or not the act is achieved, an individual survivor, having experienced mass trauma, may strive to inhabit a 'collective subject position', and thus bear witness not only for herself, but for those who cannot.

When conducting interviews with women former political prisoners in Indonesia in 2002 and 2005, it was not always clear to whom a particular woman was referring. For example, during a particular interview, a woman might begin by telling her own story of being arrested following the 1965 coup, then give details of another woman's arrest, revert back to speaking about her own experiences, and continue to intermesh the stories of other women she had known at the time with her own story. It is important to specify here that this intermeshing of experiences is by no means unproblematic.

Discursive Strategies: Contexts and Secrets

The settings for speaking are vitally important to the telling of women's narratives of genocide, torture and political imprisonment under the New Order. 'Settings' are not only the larger, sociopolitical landscape in which the women give their testimonies, but also the *mise en scène*, or sites of telling, which are 'both occasional, that is, specific to an occasion, and locational, that is, emergent in a specific . . . context of narration' (Smith and Watson 56). The how, when, where and who of these narratives are as much a part of the testimonies as the words spoken (and not spoken). As Robson has argued: 'The possibilities and limitations of language and of narrative in the face of trauma also depend on the forum in which trauma is recounted' (13).

This is because the stories told belong to the time and place in which they were told. Thus, the narrative texts presented and analysed in this project are necessarily different from those stories. The women (and men) interviewed during the course of my fieldwork in Indonesia gave testimonies as part of an interview process. By removing these oral testimonies from the interview settings in which they were told, I am aware that I often must, for the sake of the analysis, also remove the 'questions, comments, silences and exclamations that interfere, influence and help shape the testimony in its interview setting' (Unnold 117).

In particular, vital aspects of the testimonies given were the silences within those narratives and the secrets shared and not shared. As Della Pollock has argued, secrets hold the 'precarious possibility of *telling*. Whispered, half-told, announced, secrets unfold as both *risk* and *power*: as the risk of embarrassment, shame, helplessness, betrayal and judgement, and as the power of knowledge and (cabbalistic) authority' (193). During many of the interviews, for example, in often whispered conversations, narratives were told which carried with them certain risks. These risks were due to any number of complex considerations, such as feelings of shame because a certain taboo had entered into the narrative.

Sometimes the secrets shared would be those of the past. For example, one of my main contacts, Ibu Lia, who spent more than twenty years in prison, most of them in isolation, recounted a number of stories about how she and the other political prisoners in her cell block had passed hidden messages to each other. In tiny scrawl, written using hidden pencils on small, stolen pieces of paper, she and the others in the cell block would push the small messages into holes in the walls of the toilet area to communicate with one another.

On the other hand, secrets were also not shared. During any particular interview, my aim was not only to hear the narrative of a particular woman's experiences but also to explore the ways in which she told that narrative. If someone steered the conversation away from a certain topic (for whatever reason), I would not draw the conversation back to that topic. As Pollock has also argued, 'Secrecy constructs the borders it guards', thus, secrets are 'only disclosed *within* a circle of declared membership or as a means of *drawing in* the outsider, producing memberships' (186; 193). Sometimes I was drawn in to a certain extent, at other times I was most definitely left outside. As an outsider, who, on most occasions, a particular woman met only once, these negotiations of allowing me to be included or excluded in certain narratives marked different borders at different times of trust and understanding.

Particularly when the topic of sexual violence emerged, taboos were often encountered, sometimes resulting in various avoidance strategies for discussing experiences of rape and sexual assault. Here 'taboo' means 'subjects that are culturally marked as linguistically prohibitive topics of discourse' (Trinch 599). Again, in each situation, the context of narration was key. While I am not proposing that the discussion of sexual violence is marked (linguistically or otherwise) as a taboo in all parts of Indonesia or that even the ways in which it is marked are the same across the great number of ethnic and other groups there, I do want to draw attention to a few examples of occasions on which certain narrative strategies emerged when the topic of sexual violence arose.

One way a number of women negotiated these taboos discursively was by telling their own story as that of another. This narrative strategy has been studied by a number of other researchers including, for example, Vesna Nikolic-Ristanovic, whose work has examined gendered violence against women during the conflict in the former Yugoslavia and Kosovo in the 1990s. As in the Nikolic-Ristanovic study, I found that third person narratives would emerge, telling the story of what happened to a 'friend' or to another woman/women in the same cell or the same camp (207). It was also not uncommon for a woman to talk about 'all the women', referring to either 'everyone in the cell with me', 'all the women in the same camp/prison' or 'all the women in this region'. As Nikolic-Ristanovic found, one reason for employing these discursive strategies may have been to avoid the stigmatisation that is often associated with victims of sexual assault (24). Another reason may have been that the experiences recounted were traumatic and difficult to narrate. One example of this was during an interview with three women (Ibu Sri, Ibu Lani and Ibu Nana) who were all from the same region in Sumatra. We had been discussing what had happened during the killings and mass arrests in that area when Ibu Nana and Ibu Lani, together, told this story:

> **Ibu Lani:** There were many women who were taken as wives because their husbands had been taken, so the wives would be taken. Then they'd be gang raped, one after another. There was lots of that! In [this region] there were only three of us. Three of us who weren't ...
>
> **Ibu Nana:** Who weren't raped.
>
> **Ibu Lani:** This woman [she is referring to herself] and one other.
>
> **Ibu Nana:** She was old, even the older women were raped.
>
> **Ibu Lani:** Raped! The only reason I wasn't raped was because I had only recently given birth. [I had been] pregnant. So wherever I was interrogated, I held my baby to me. I held on, so they wouldn't take the baby from me. But if I hadn't had my baby with me, I would have been ... (pauses) sexually assaulted ... we couldn't do anything. We couldn't fight back.
>
> **Annie:** If someone fought back ...?
>
> **Ibu Lani:** They'd be shot ... We'd be brought [for interrogation], but the weapon that I had was the little baby that I had. That was the only thing I had. [...] Really, there were only three in [this region]. For the whole of [this region], only three weren't raped. (Pauses) The others, well ...

Another discursive strategy which appeared was the use of euphemisms and ambiguous or vague terms to refer to different actions or events during sexual assaults. In her analysis of lexical variants used by Latina women to describe sexual violence, Shonna L. Trinch found that 'the use of terminology that palliates indecency and indelicacy in order to uphold decorum plays a key role in the construction of sexual assault narratives' (572). Euphemisms are therefore employed and, as Charles Kany found, are 'the means by which a disagreeable, offensive, or fear-instilling matter is designated with an indirect or softer term. Euphemisms satisfy a linguistic need. For his own sake as well as that of his listeners, a speaker constantly resorts to euphemism in order to disguise an unpleasant truth, veil an offence, or palliate indecency' (v). Trinch argues that these strategies are 'manipulated by speakers to avoid loss of face or to offer to their interlocutors, as well as to guard for themselves, *a way out* of a potentially offensive interpretation of an utterance' (571).

The following example is taken from an interview with Ibu Eny who was relating incidents of sexual assault during the killings and interrogations. My contact in that area, Narny Yenny, had previously interviewed Ibu Eny on a number of occasions as part of her own research and, as is clear in the text, begins by prompting her to tell a particular story. In this example, I want to draw attention to the omission of verb subjects (perpetrators in particular), and the use of more ambiguous verbs in place of verbs which describe specific actions. Examples in the following text of these ambiguous verbs are '*di(be)ginikan*' and '*digitukan*' which follow the passive construction '*di*—base verb—*kan*'; '*gini*' and '*gitu*', in this case, roughly meaning 'like this' or 'like that', creating passive verbs meaning something approximating 'an action that was done by someone/ something else to someone/something'. Gestures and bodily actions were used together with these verbally ambiguous descriptions to create a much more clear, embodied narrative performance.

> **Upik:** *Bu*, about the sexual abuse ...
>
> **Ibu Eny:** Oh, [you mean] if there was anyone raped?
>
> **Upik:** Yes. Just about that, *Bu*.
>
> **Ibu Eny:** Those who were raped, they weren't with me. I was in prison when it happened.
>
> **Upik:** But you had to take off your clothes ...?
>
> **Ibu Eny:** Yes, when [we] were questioned/interrogated, [we] had to take off [our] clothes.
>
> **Upik:** You had your clothes removed ...
>
> **Ibu Eny:** Everything was taken off ... yes, me and the other women [with me] all had our clothes taken off, [...]. Yes, taken off, they said because they wanted to check for tattoos, if [you were in] Gerwani (one of the Indonesian Communist Party's associated organisations), a Gerwani tattoo, if [you were in] Pemuda Rakyat (the Communist Party's youth organisation), [then] a Pemuda Rakyat tattoo would be looked for [...] Everything was taken off. Naked. That's what it was like for us [...] the same again at the military station and at the police station [where they] did the interrogations. [There were] three who faced us.
>
> **Annie**: Men?
>
> **Ibu Eny:** Men. At the time [when we had to] take off our clothes, [we] didn't want to be beaten. Yes, we were ordered to stand up, all our clothes were taken down, only our underpants were left. Ha, it was like that that we were inspected. Our breasts, *ni*, *diginikan* (she clutches at her own breasts, pulling them up forcefully) to the top, they said there was a tattoo there. Ha, there's a tattoo here (she lifts her sarong with one hand, the other grabs the front of her underpants), they said there's a tattoo here. In reality, I think, it wasn't a tattoo but our privates that [they] were looking at, like that. One person would have been checked and of course there wouldn't be any [tattoos]. There weren't any, but we were all *digitukan* [treated in this manner].

Testimonio, Post-Suharto Indonesia and Talking about 1965

Beverley, in addressing the problematic relationship between *testimonio* and truth, draws our attention to the original Spanish—*dar testimonio* or 'to give testimony', which, as he says, 'carries the connotation of an act of truth telling in a religious or legal sense ... [it] means to testify, to bear truthful witness' (*Testimonio* 3). Yet *testimonio* is not, nor was it ever intended to be, legal testimony—in the sense that it is not the testimony given by a witness in a courtroom with the evidence in that testimony governed by a particular body of rules determining its admissibility. But as *testimonio* is removed from the 'category of truth produced by legal discourse' (Gilmore, 'Jurisdictions' 699), the consequences of this removal must also be considered. In particular, the question is, how do these consequences affect the survivors, such as Ibu Eny, whose stories are told in post-Suharto Indonesia about the killings and mass detentions following the 1965 coup?

Given that this kind of testimony 'does not conceive of itself as legal testimony, and thus does not constitute ... legal fact' (Weine 23), this unavoidably means that such testimony cannot be used 'as is' in any legal system. Nor does it fulfil the requirements of admissible evidence that would be necessary for prosecuting perpetrators of these crimes. Yet to uncover and redress the human rights' abuses committed under the New Order regime since the fall of Suharto, non-legal avenues must be pursued. *Testimonio* raises issues of truth, truth-telling, multiple subjectivities and the situations of urgency and trauma from which they emerge, and yet despite these dilemmas (or, in fact, because of them), *testimonio* offers a political and analytical framework with which to collect, analyse and circulate survivors' narratives.

With the creation of a Truth and Reconciliation Commission in Indonesia at a standstill, there is also an urgency for this process to begin—not only because an official investigation into the killings and other human rights' abuses is long overdue but also because the survivors of those abuses are running out of time. The youngest woman former political prisoner with whom I spoke was in her late fifties, the eldest in her mid-nineties. Given the failure of successive governments since the fall of the New Order in 1998 to carry out official investigations into the events of 1965, the testimonies of those who survived these events must find other avenues for documentation and circulation while survivors remain to testify.

Notes

[1] 'Ibu Eny' is a pseudonym for a woman I interviewed in September 2005 in Sumatra, Indonesia. 'Ibu' is a term of address for older, usually married, women in Indonesia. All names, places and other identifying information have been erased or obscured.

[2] The precise number of people murdered and imprisoned following the 1 October 1965 alleged Communist coup is unknown. For further information about the coup, the killings of 1965–66 and mass political imprisonments, see key works by Benedict R. Anderson and Ruth T. McVey, Robert Cribb, and Justus M. van der Kroef listed in the References.

[3] See those works by Saskia Wieringa and Steven Drakeley.
[4] Interview with Pak I___, Central Java, November 2005.
[5] The case was rejected by the Central Jakarta District Court in September of that year. See Ima (n.p.).
[6] Interview with Ibu A___, Jakarta, October 2005.
[7] See, for example, those works by H. D. Haryo Sasongko and Melanie Budianta, John Roosa, Ayu Ratih and Hilmar Farid, and Asvi Warman Adam. By 'widely available' I mean that if one were to go into a Gramedia store (Indonesia's largest bookstore chain), such books are available. However, comparatively, books are quite expensive for the general population despite rampant copyright infingements and mass photocopying, so by 'widely available' I mean 'easily available to those with adequate funds and access, usually those in the middle class and above'. Also, it must be said that there was also a handful of works published in the last years of Suharto's regime which contradicted the New Order government's version of the 1965 events, such as *Bayang-Bayang PKI* [Shadows of the Indonesian Communist Party] by ISAI, the Institute for the Studies on Free Flow of Information, in 1995.
[8] My use of the term 'prototype' here refers to categorisation theory, see George Lakoff and Mark Johnson (19–20).

References

A___, Ibu. Personal Interview. Oct. 2005.

Adam, Asvi Warman. *Soeharto: Sisi Gelap Sejarah Indonesia* [Suharto: The Dark Side of Indonesian History]. Yogyakarta: Ombak, 2004.

Anderson, Benedict R, and Ruth T. McVey. *A Preliminary Analysis of the October 1, 1965, Coup in Indonesia*. Ithaca: Cornell UP, 1971.

Beverley, John. 'The Margin at the Center: On Testimonio (Testimonial Narrative).' *Modern Fiction Studies* 35.1 (1989): 11–28.

——. *Testimonio: On the Politics of Truth*. Minneapolis: U of Minnesota P, 2004.

Cribb, Robert, ed. *The Indonesian Killings of 1965–1966: Studies from Java and Bali*. Clayton, VIC: Centre of Southeast Asian Studies, Monash U, 1990.

Delbo, Charlotte. *Mesure de Nos Jours*. Paris: Minuit, 1971.

Des Pres, Terrence. *The Survivor: An Anatomy of Life in the Death Camps*. New York: Oxford UP, 1976.

Drakeley, Steven. *Lubang Buaya: Myth, Misogyny, and Massacre*. Clayton, VIC: Centre for Southeast Asian Studies, 2000.

Eny, Ibu. Personal Interview. Sept. 2005.

Flanagan, Patrick, and Julie Southwood. *Indonesia: Law, Propaganda and Terror*. London: Zed Books, 1983.

Gilmore, Leigh. 'Jurisdictions: *I, Rigoberta Menchu*, *The Kiss*, and Scandalous Self-Representation in the Age of Memoir and Trauma.' *Signs* 28.2 (2003): 695–718.

——. *The Limits of Autobiography: Trauma and Testimony*. Ithaca: Cornell UP, 2001.

Heryanto, Ariel. 'Where Communism Never Dies: Violence, Trauma and Narration in the Last Cold War Capitalist Authoritarian State.' *International Journal of Cultural Studies* 2.2 (1999): 147–77.

I___, Pak. Personal Interview. Nov. 2005.

Ima. 'Majelis Hakim PN Jakpus Tolak Gugatan Korban Stigma PKI.' *Kompas* 14 Sept. 2005. 10 March 2007. <http://www.kompas.com/utama/news/0509/14/145639.htm>.

Tapol. *Indonesia: The Prison State*. London: Tapol, 1976.

ISAI [Institute for the Studies on Free Flow of Information]. *Bayang-Bayang PKI*. Jakarta: ISAI, 1995.

Kany, Charles. *American Spanish Euphemisms*. Berkeley: U of California P, 1960.
Kearney, Marianne. 'Oppressed Writer Sues President.' *The Courier-Mail* 16 March 2005: 21.
van der Kroef, Justus M. 'Indonesia's Political Prisoners.' *Pacific Affairs* 49 (1976): 625–47.
Lakoff, George, and Mark Johnson. *Philosophy in the Flesh: The Embodied Mind and its Challenges to Western Thought*. New York: Basic Books, 1999.
Lani, Ibu. Personal Interview. Sept. 2005.
Menchu, Rigoberta. *I, Rigoberta Menchu—An Indian Woman in Guatemala*. Ed. Elisabeth Burgos-Debray. Trans. Ann Wright. London: Verso, 1984.
Nana, Ibu. Personal Interview. Sept. 2005.
Nikolic-Ristanovic, Vesna, ed. *Women, Violence and War: Wartime Victimization of Refugees in the Balkans*. Budapest: Central European UP, 1999.
Pollock, Della. *Telling Bodies, Performing Birth: Everyday Narratives of Childbirth*. New York: Columbia UP, 1999.
Rice-Sayre, L. P. 'Witnessing History: Diplomacy Versus *Testimony*.' *Testimonio y Literatura*. Ed. R. a. H. V. Jara. Minneapolis: Society for the Study of Contemporary Hispanic and Lusophone Revolutionary Literatures, 1986. 48–72.
Robson, Kathryn. *Writing Wounds: The Inscription of Trauma in Post-1968 French Women's Life-Writing*. Amsterdam: Rodopi, 2004.
Roosa, John, Ayu Ratih, and Hilmar Farid, eds. *Tahun yang Tak Pernah Berakhir: Memahami Pengalaman Korban. '65* [The Year that Never Ended: Understanding the Experiences of the '65 Victims]. Jakarta: ELSAM, TruK and ISSI, 2004.
Sanford, Victoria. *Buried Secrets: Truth and Human Rights in Guatemala*. New York: Palgrave MacMillan, 2003.
Sasongko, H. D. Haryo, and Melanie Budianta, eds. *Menembus Tirai Asap: Kesaksian Tahanan Politik 1965* [Piercing the Smoke Screen: Witness Accounts by the 1965 Political Prisoners]. Jakarta: Amanah-Lontar, 2003.
Schaffer, Kay, and Sidonie Smith. 'Conjunctions: Life Narratives in the Field of Human Rights.' *Biography* 27.1 (2004): 1–24.
Smith, Sidonie, and Julia Watson. *Reading Autobiography: A Guide for Interpreting Life Narratives*. Minneapolis: U of Minnesota P, 2001.
Sommer, Dorris. '"Not Just a Personal Story": Women's Testimonios and the Plural Self.' *Life/Lines: Theorizing Women's Autobiography*. Ed. Bella and Celeste Schenck Brodski. Ithaca: Cornell UP, 1988. 107–30.
Sri, Ibu. Personal Interview. Sept. 2005.
Stoler, Ann Laura. 'On the Uses and Abuses of the Past in Indonesia.' *Asian Survey* 42.4 (2002): 642–50.
Stoll, David. *Rigoberta Menchu and the Story of All Poor Guatemalans*. Boulder: Westview P, 1999.
Trinch, Shonna L. 'Managing Euphemism and Transcending Taboos: Negotiating the Meaning of Sexual Assault in Latinas. Narratives of Domestic Violence.' *Text* 21.4 (2001): 567–610.
Unnold, Yvonne S. *Representing the Unrepresentable: Literature of Trauma under Pinochet in Chile*. New York: Lang, 2002.
Weine, Stevan. *Testimony After Catastrophe: Narrating the Traumas of Political Violence*. Evanston, IL: Northwestern UP, 2006.
Whitlock, Gillian. *The Intimate Empire: Reading Women's Autobiography*. London: Cassell, 2000.
Wieringa, Saskia. *Sexual Politics in Indonesia*. New York: Palgrave, 2002.
Yudice, Georg. 'Testimonio and Postmodernism.' *Latin American Perspectives* 70.18.3 (1991): 15–31.
Zurbuchen, Mary S. 'History, Memory, and the "1965 Incident" in Indonesia.' *Asian Survey* 42.4 (2002): 564–82.

Fifty Years On: Melancholic (Re)collections and Women's Voices from the Partition of India

Terri Tomsky

In her historiographical study, *The Other Side of Silence* (2000), Urvashi Butalia writes about the oddly unnerving experience of interviewing the survivors of the 1947 Indian partition, 'witnesses' for whom memories of partition prompt 'bitterness, rage, and hatred—which, once uncovered, could be frightening' (5).[1] That these fifty-year old memories can trigger the immediacy and anguish of partition tells us something about the lack of closure surrounding the event.

But at the same time, it is important to consider how the emotions produced by the testimonies affect the interviewer, literally frightening her. Here the past erupts into the present as the act of testimony reconstitutes and transfers the trauma of partition violence. Butalia's experience appears to be an excellent example of the power of narratives circulating in what Sara Ahmed has called an 'affective economy'. For Ahmed, affect acts as a transferential, contagious force, shaping individual and collective bodies across time (*Cultural Politics* 15). Butalia's autobiographical confession, amidst her scholarly introduction to the study, reveals the way emotions and the experiential are *formative*, the way they articulate her subject position as an academic writer and historian. The implications of this emotional charge are severe, especially if we consider that the traditional imperative for the scholar-editor is to remain as dispassionate and disinterested as possible. Butalia seems to recognise this as she attends to the disjuncture between her affectively-charged experience and the absence of affect in official historical documentations of partition. As she notes, emotions such as 'loss', 'joy and grief', and 'painful regret and nostalgia' are 'difficult things to capture "factually". Yet, could it really be that they had no place in the history of Partition?' (6). Butalia's unsettling experience is not unique among recent partition scholarship. Many editors, historians, interviewers, and critics palpably bear the effects of this emotional transference in their writing.

This essay tries to answer Butalia's question by demonstrating the centrality of affect in shaping the subjective position of the partition scholar, the figure who tries to make sense of the lingering or unresolved legacy of India's traumatic partition. For the most part, I will confine my argument to the relationship between affect, life narratives, and the emerging genre of literary partition anthologies. The partition anthology is an Indian genre that establishes dialogues with an English-speaking readership and the Indian nation-state. Published in English on the Indian subcontinent, these anthologies focus on the partition through a series of literary and/or autobiographical narratives. Such anthologies first appeared in 1976, and have steadily grown in number. Generically, anthologies are important not only because their use of multiple narratives makes them appear more 'representative' and able to encase a collective or national trauma, but also because they remain implicated in pedagogical institutions, especially universities.[2] The partition anthologies are predominantly literary collections, mainly short stories, rather than collections of testimony or life narratives.[3] Nevertheless, they offer an autobiographical peritext that frames the anthology and that shapes its scholarship.[4] So while the anthologies are dominated by literary texts, the focal point in this essay will be the anthological editor who finds his or her critical voice both constrained and directed by their encounter with traumatic affect.

To understand how affect structures the autobiographical editorial voice, it is first necessary to clarify what I mean by the term. Broadly speaking, 'affect' describes an emotional force, relating both to sensation and to an intensity of feeling, which compels or inspires a subject to (re)act in the world. Current theories of affect diverge from this basic point of departure but, as Nigel Thrift has shown, among them is a consensus that affect is 'a form of thinking, often indirect and non-reflective ... but thinking all the same' (60). Affect theory opens a way to release emotion from the prisonhouse of the Cartesian mind/body split. It need no longer be hermetically sealed away from rational or objective calculations, nor need it be understood as supplementary to thought. Via affect theory, certain strong feelings are reconfigured as the agents rather than as the catalysts of knowledge production. In this sense, affect obtains a political dimension, a worldliness, and as Thrift continues, 'attempts which have relegated affect to the irrational or raised it up to the level of the sublime are both equally wrong-headed' (60).

If we return to Butalia's question of whether it is possible to register the emotions of partition trauma as facts, which could eventually be used to unsettle existing state narratives of the event, we see how affective politics offers a tentative resolution. In this paper, I am concerned with the role of melancholia as an affect that dominates partition scholarship and, particularly, that emerges in the editorial practices connected to the production of partition anthologies. What I want to suggest is that melancholia does not simply indicate that the editors are all too human, or that melancholia is something that must be overcome if we ever hope to speak critically about the partition experience. Rather melancholia, as an affect, plays a *critical* role in the production of knowledge and especially in the positioning of the anthological editor as a legitimate knowledge producer. The editor, through his or her autobiographical peritext, 'charges' the anthology (as an object). Once the anthology is an affectively-charged object it can, to return to Ahmed's concept, circulate and transfer to its reader; the affective economy expands with each new transaction. The political point becomes clear if we realise that the effect of the anthology on the reader is similar to that of those testimonies which an interviewer like Butalia found so disturbing. The purpose of affectively-charged anthologies is thus to trouble the reader, simultaneously to constrain and direct a new response to a past trauma made present once again.

This essay considers the mobilisation of melancholic affect in two types of anthologies. The first case occurs in the most popular type, the anthology of partition literature. Here the purpose is to identify the way editing, understood as the attempt to cultivate a cultural narrative of partition, is a product not only of a professional but also of a personal desire to speak about partition traumas. To elaborate this, I consider two representative anthologies. The first, Alok Bhalla's *Stories about the Partition of India* (1994), is widely recognised as the most comprehensive anthology of partition literature to date. The second, Debjani Sengupta's *Mapmaking: Partition Stories From 2 Bengals* (2003), is an excellent example of the second-wave of partition anthologies, which are distinguished by their attention to regional or minority accounts of the partition experience. For both editors, it is clear that the drive towards creating a partition anthology is overdetermined by their respective desires to write of their personal history. The second part of the analysis turns away from literary anthologies to consider instead a recent collection of partition testimonies, Ritu

Menon's *No Woman's Land: Women from Pakistan, India, and Bangladesh Write on the Partition of India* (2004). Whereas literary editors tend to subordinate life writing to literary works—and sometimes do so explicitly—Menon's anthology harnesses the powerful affect contained in women's testimonies in order to generate a feminist critique of the existing hegemonic interpretation of the events of 1947.

To apprehend the political dimension of affect in both cases, we need to understand how the post-partition states responded to the traumatic event, both in their material practices and in their hegemonic historiography. Like the Nazi Holocaust, the legacies of partition are profound and catastrophic, with generations today still grappling with how to remember the event. The partitioning of India along communal lines displaced some twelve million people, killed at least a million, and involved mass abductions and the mutilation of women.[5] The communal hatred and gratuitous brutality of partition shattered both society and the self. For example, in her work on Urdu writer Saadat Hasan Manto, Priyamvada Gopal identifies the extent of the trauma when she notes that partition left 'reverberations of ... communal hatred and bloodshed ... the wounded recesses where the individual and community colluded in doing violence to themselves and to others in the cause of self-assertion' (91).

The mourning of partition's victims and the working through of its manifold violences and losses have yet to be achieved. Primarily this is because the outcome of partition was the 'birth' of the states of India and Pakistan (and later, Bangladesh). Instead of acknowledging the trauma, or commemorating the suffering of partition, these new nations focused on the triumph of Independence over the colonial past. Yet in a seminal study of trauma and historiography, Dominick LaCapra argues that, '[s]omething of the past always remains, if only as a haunting presence' (49). We can apply LaCapra's observation to the 'haunting presence' of memories and affect that make themselves felt in Butalia's interviews. Sigmund Freud's theorisation of melancholia is useful for thinking about survivors' experience of partition years later. In his 1915 essay, 'Mourning and Melancholia', Freud distinguished between mourning and melancholia as two opposite modes (one healthy, the other unhealthy), which dealt with a subject's attachment to what Freud termed the 'lost object' (244). In mourning, the past has elapsed and is considered finished; melancholia, in contrast, can be understood as a clinging to the past through this lost object. In their study on loss and mourning, David Eng and David Kazanjian note that melancholia involves 'an ongoing and open relationship with the past—bringing its ghosts and spectres, its flaring and fleeting images into the present' (4). In other words, melancholia signifies a compression of time between the present and the traumatic past, in which the past intrudes into the present.

I want to break with the Freudian concept of 'good' mourning versus 'bad' melancholia to consider briefly the way melancholia has been theorised recently as a critical force. For instance, LaCapra talks about a 'melancholic sentiment', a 'bond with the dead' that can enable 're-engagement in life' (22). Similarly, Eng and Kazanjian see a 'continuous engagement' with the losses of the past as positive since it 'generates sites for memory and history, for the rewriting of the past as well as the reimagining of the future' (4). This kind of productive melancholic attachment to the past has been explicated elsewhere by Ahmed and Eric Santner amongst others; I see one such iteration of melancholia in partition scholarship and the narratives of cultural productions. Scholars such as Joe Cleary, Jill Didur, and Ananya Kabir have called attention to the central role of partition narratives in recuperating and disseminating traumatic memories. In particular, the refusal to 'let go' of the past, in order to retain and delineate partition's traumas, is what makes thinking about these texts and their authors in terms of melancholia useful.

Whereas Cleary, Didur, and Kabir concentrate on novels and short stories in their discussions of collective cultural memories, it seems to me that we have overlooked the significance of the anthology, a genre in many ways *designed* to articulate a collective voice. The very growth of this genre implies on the one hand a proverbial 'gap' in the scholarship, a need to revisit the partition in order to explore more fully the contours of its traumas. At the same time the growth both reflects and accelerates developments in a public, collective consciousness about partition. Though there have always existed various forms of consciousness about partition, the emergence of partition anthologies, as with literary works and partition scholarship, indicates a public readiness for a wider discussion and acknowledgement about the event and its effects.

These anthologies are especially significant because of their specific institutional affiliations. Long understood as a pedagogical genre, anthologies consolidate canons and cultural traditions and, in the Indian context, partition anthologies have the ability to establish partition as a topic of importance and contribute to the formations of a national consciousness and debate about partition memory. In her work on ethnic anthologies, the Canadian writer and critic Smaro Kamboureli describes the critical, cultural, and pedagogic role of anthologies when she explains that, by their very structure and subject, anthologies are designed to 'make a collective statement' (133). Because they so often include academic introductions and other critical editorial paratextual material, anthologies offer a self-conscious mode of articulating and institutionalising a distinctly collective trauma. As such, anthologies can remedy what Ritu Menon and Kamla Bhasin identify as the 'paucity of social histories' of the Indian partition (6), by calling attention to existing testimonies or standing in for absent life-narratives since 'the overwhelming majority of [partition's] events went unrecorded, [and] unverbalised' (7). More readily than a single text, anthologies assert a range of partition experiences, conveying the scope and significance of the Indian partition in terms of its considerable historical repercussions and its traumas.[6] As Kay Schaffer and Sidonie Smith point out in their 2004 study of testimony and human rights, breadth and diversity perform an important function in motivating the reader politically: 'anthologies gain their ethical force by gathering multiple narratives of shared victimization into one volume whose purpose is to challenge and rewrite history, call the reader to recognition, and spur action' (45).

The emergence of the partition anthology does signal important shifts in the public recognition of partition's traumatic legacies; in this genre, editors contribute to the process of rewriting contemporary Indian history and demanding recognition within a national context that has hitherto lacked public commemoration of the suffering experienced. However, while these anthologies are designed to represent a collective, they contain at their core the personal experiences and memories of individual intellectuals, the figures who are instrumental in their compilation.[7] Indeed, in many cases, the editors do not hide this personal interest but rather often ponder the nature of the relationship between their personal memories and their scholarly pursuits. Consider once more Butalia's anecdote about the disturbance produced by her proximity (in the role of a compiler) to the traumatic experiences of people unknown to her. For Butalia, this cross-generational affect is both distinct from and more powerful than the partition memories she inherited from her family. Yet at the same time, she seems keen to explore the relation between the affect of her scholarly experience and her inherited memories: 'Ever since I can remember we had heard stories of Partition', she admits, but then adds that it was only as she worked and spoke with victims of the 1984 reprisals against the Sikh community (following the assassination of Indira Gandhi) that the 'stories of Partition no longer seemed so remote' (Butalia 4).

The productive exchange between (a scholar's) personal autobiography and their experience in handling, selecting, and organising partition texts characterises not only Butalia's historiographical study, but also partition anthologies. Even while many anthology editors prefer to attempt to 'represent' the partition experience through selections of short stories and poetry, their autobiographical voice cannot be overlooked. Consider, for instance, *the* pre-eminent (in terms of size, scope, and critical acclaim) partition anthology, Bhalla's *Stories about the Partition of India*, which argues that literary narratives, rather than life writings, function as 'appalled witnesses to an age of genocide' (xviii). While Bhalla privileges the literary and the aesthetic in his attempt to initiate 'an ethical inquiry' into the violence of partition and ongoing communalism, it is his *personal memories* of partition that saturate the peritext (x). In his introduction, for example, in contrast to the institutional celebratory rhetoric surrounding Independence, Bhalla asserts an experience of crisis: 'my childhood consciousness was scarred by the cruelties I saw during the riots of 1947–48 and the lamentations I heard' (x). Bhalla's autobiographical account provides a form of witnessing that intersects with the fictional stories of his anthology in his narration of loss and suffering. Haunted by his 'earliest memory', Bhalla recalls a nameless Muslim trader who had been sheltered by his father during one of partition's many riots (x). The man had initially left Bhalla's house safely but, later seeing a mob, had tried to turn back. When Bhalla unlocks the door a few hours later, he recalls the sight of a 'body of a man ... [his] limbs in disarray, his clothes ... soaked in blood' on the doorstep (x). For Bhalla, the trauma of this incident is seared deeply into his mind: 'I have never since forgotten that day' (xi). Indeed, we can see in Bhalla's frequent references to communal violence as 'inexplicable', 'evil', 'madness' that creates 'utter bewilderment', reflections of his own disorientation and traumatised memory, from which he cannot distance himself (xi; xxiv; ix).

The presence of Bhalla's autobiography in the editorial introduction is not simply meant to justify his subjective position. Rather, like his decision to collate three volumes, totalling sixty-three stories on partition, he sees his personal testimony as representative of something larger. As he explains:

> Over the years, I came to realize that my recollections of those days were not private ... Similar incidents were known to others and had become a part of their experiential world. My own memories began to acquire a density and a detail from the narratives of a variety of different people. (Bhalla xi)

Bhalla's autobiographical reminiscences illustrate the processes in which a collective trauma accumulates from manifold memories about partition, creating the 'density' and 'detail' of a larger experience. His life narrative consequently works in tandem with the collected pieces of fiction; together, they assert partition as 'the single most traumatic experience in our recent history' (vii). The collective formation of trauma is not only made up of the traumatic memories and stories but, as with Butalia's accounts, also registers the haunting affects of partition, the 'anger and grief' of passers-by and victims, the 'guilt' and the 'remorse' of perpetrators (xv). It is clear that, in partition anthologies, fiction and autobiography neither occupy separate spaces, nor utilise separate vocabularies, nor communicate emotions in different ways. Both are bound together, and in this way they are both intimately yet differently engaged in the memory work of partition narratives.

An affective crossover between the (editorial) personal and the (authorial) fictional also takes place in Sengupta's partition anthology, *Mapmaking*. Like Bhalla, Sengupta prefers short stories to illustrate the different traumatic memories of partition, although *Mapmaking* is much smaller, comprising only ten short stories and focusing on the regional experience of partition in Bengal and Bangladesh. But even so, *Mapmaking* remains enmeshed in the familial memories of its editor, Sengupta, and the author of its foreword, Ashis Nandy. For her part, Sengupta relays a second-generation consciousness that is founded upon her parents' recollections of a lost Home. The child of East Bengali migrants that came to what was then Calcutta (now Kolkata), Sengupta dedicates her anthology to her parents for passing on their 'memories of East Bengal'. This dedication attests to a melancholic and exilic longing for the 'lost' other. It suggests that the other Bengal continues to function as an imaginary homeland, an affective site of desire, loss, and unattainability that haunts the East Bengali migrant generations. Though she avoids any further reference to her personal entanglement in the history of partition, Sengupta's argument that the Bengal partition involves an ongoing 'metaphysical [hurt] ... in the mind, the soul' suggests that the trauma of partition is inextricable from the personal, as it remains embodied in the self (188).

For Sengupta, partition is construed as the catastrophe of Bengali identity; yet she also suggests that the memory of this trauma will draw the two Bengals together again. To reflect the promise of this reunion, Sengupta uses bodily metaphors to structure our understanding of Bengali territory. This governing metaphor is elaborated as she posits East and West Bengal as codependent bodily parts. Taking as its signal note Subhas Mukhopadhyay's poem, 'Ferrying', *Mapmaking* is a study of the cultures of the two Bengals, which are 'like the two pupils/of the eyes of Bangladesh' (Sengupta 186).[8] Thus rather than interpreting (Indian) West Bengal and (Pakistani/Bangladeshi) East Bengal as discrete lenses, the metaphor implies a degree of similarity. Each eye will see, in the final analysis, practically the same thing; at most, their difference is of the slightest perspective; what remains behind the eyes is a central nervous system, a shared brain that processes the data into meaning.

Through the partition anthologies edited by Bhalla and Sengupta, we are privy to previously private forms of collective consciousness about partition: the memories of family and friends that have not been part of the public sphere to date. These have circulated in the private sphere where they are sustained as popular memories about lived experience that are passed down orally, transgenerationally, and mediated within social institutions like the family, where they persist as rumours, sentiment, or what Marianne Hirsch calls 'postmemory'. First developed in *Family Frames: Photography, Narrative, and Postmemory* (1997), Hirsch's concept describes the way traumatic memories transfer affect across generations. Hirsch herself concentrates on photographs, whose power comes from their status as objects that 'carry an emotional weight especially in the face of the monumental losses' (14). In a more recent essay, Hirsch narrows her definition of postmemory to mean, quite specifically, 'the response of the second generation to the trauma of the first' ('of ... Monumental losses' 8). Her clarification is useful for elaborating notions of bearing witness through the formation of an affective relationship between the past and the present. Nevertheless, in limiting her analysis to family lines, Hirsch's theory also circumscribes the complex ways by which an original and traumatic memory haunts future generations as postmemories. Certainly Bhalla's narrative indicates some form of postmemory as he recuperates his experience of trauma through the collective and haunting memories of others, so many years later. Likewise, in the case of Butalia, it is not her personal familial memories of partition, but rather her professional experience with witnesses that spurs the exchange of traumatic affect. In both cases, it appears that these postmemories are then carried into future generations through the circuit of partition scholarship.

In his foreword to *Mapmaking*, Nandy draws the reader's attention to affective haunting in partition writing. Nandy, a political psychologist and sociologist, turns to theories of the Freudian repressed in order to understand how the 'past traumata of a collectivity',

> haunt[s] not only the direct victims and the perpetrators, but also the following generations, which inherit without as much as an exchange of a word on the subject, the fears, the anxieties, tensions ... [the] unexamined past has to be lived out over the succeeding generations. (ix)

By positioning partition as a repressed event around which the social and cultural fabric of India is constituted, the affects of partition trauma constitute a haunting return—a return that is, in part, mediated by these anthologies. The diffusion of affect within communities, groups, and families, as described by Nandy, is consonant with Ranjana Khanna's recent theorisation of melancholia and its haunting symptoms in *Dark Continents: Psychoanalysis and Colonialism* (2003). Khanna's theory, building on Freud as well as the work of psychoanalytic scholars Nicholas Abraham and Maria Torok, reformulates melancholia as an ambivalent dynamic of loss *and* critical agency. She argues that when a trauma occurs and is repressed, it fails to be assimilated, *pace* Freud's theories of unsuccessful mourning in 'Mourning and Melancholia'. For Khanna, the inassimilable remainder of a repressed trauma manifests as a resonant melancholia; the symptoms of melancholia appear as haunting through language and discourses, as affect that is passed down through generations. In Nandy's description of partition, the trauma is repressed rather than worked through, which means that negative affects are passed onto future generations. The disavowal of the root cause of bad or traumatic feelings leads to a cycle of violence, a volatile resurfacing of affect, manifested in riots and communal violence.[9] By viewing the stories of *Mapmaking* as a 'pervasive melancholia that comes from a cramping sense of guilt', Nandy reiterates Khanna's central point, that melancholia not only emerges as a haunting, but also manifests itself in language and discourses (viii). Nandy implies the critical agency at play within melancholia when he argues that *Mapmaking*'s stories antagonise the readers, and consequently provoke them into finding out 'their political and moral inheritance' (xi). For while this unsettling is partially intended to agitate the reader by foregrounding his or her complicity in the continued repression of trauma, it also suggests how a collective (the readership) might use this unsettling to interrogate the established state-level narrative of the events of 1947. Thus melancholia does not stultify but actually energises, becoming the agent for remedial anti-state activity.

A third collection, Menon's anthology of women's life writing, more directly demonstrates how melancholia can be cultivated and deployed. Gathering sixteen interviews, anecdotes, and life writings, *No Woman's Land* should be read as part of Menon's larger project to rehabilitate life writing within partition studies. In tandem with her scholarly monograph, *Borders and Boundaries: Women in India's Partition* (1998), co-authored with Kamla Bhasin, *No Woman's Land* purposes to explode the unwillingness among scholars to accredit testimony as a legitimate mode for understanding the historical and cultural implications of partition. Both these texts investigate the phenomenon of communal honour killings, the Indian government's recovery of abducted women, and the rehabilitation of dislocated women. Using short testimonial excerpts, *Borders and Boundaries* identifies the limits of existing historiography when it applies a critical feminist framework to partition. The anthology makes the complementary move, using the genre's pedagogical influence to place women's life narratives squarely within the 'canon' of partition scholarship.

The shift to the partition anthology genre for *No Woman's Land* is a strategic decision on Menon's part that calls into question both the traditional forms and authorship of partition's cultural history. In adding women's testimonies to the dialogue formulated by partition anthologies, Menon builds upon existing feminist partition scholarship, while also challenging the work produced thus far. Reflecting on the generic character of anthologies, Kamboureli has suggested that anthologies, 'perhaps more than individual titles, reflect the values shaping a given tradition'; conversely, the emergence of new anthologies like Menon's indicates, 'a perceived need to revise that tradition' (133). As with autobiographies and literary works on partition, partition anthologies register cultural narratives as alternative forms of partition history; but because many of these texts have been written by men, they also replicate the male account of partition as normative. In *No Woman's Land*, Menon castigates these works for being 'mostly fictional, mostly male', with 'little attempt to present cross-border accounts that are experiential' or to provide 'a gendered perspective' of partition (2).[10] For Menon, then, the shift to life narrative allows women's experiences to assume their proper place in the formulation of cultural memories of partition.

In introducing an array of women's experiences, *No Woman's Land* claims to illuminate a central but thus-far repressed historical event, namely that the 'real work of rehabilitating women fell to women' (8). If Menon's turn to women's life writing demonstrates the need to supplement the literary narratives used by previous anthologies, it also serves to underline the validity of women's experiences as historical accounts. Menon contests the idea that women are 'presumed to be outside history because they are outside the public and the political, where history is made' (3). She instead emphasises a feminist historiography through quotidian life. According to Menon, it is 'in women's experience, [that] the personal is the political' (3); here, the 'dailiness of [female] lives' produces 'that forgotten dimension of history in which differences are forgiven and hostilities are buried' (4). If Menon's focus on the everyday calls attention to undervalued groups, it also offers an alternative view of historiography. Her work resonates with Didur's insistence on the need to privilege '"the particular" rather than "the general" in an effort to disrupt the state's universalising and hegemonic historic narratives' (42). For Menon, women's autobiographies unsettle accepted historical and cultural discourses of 'nation and religion, community and identity ... shame and honour, blood and belonging' (10). By utilising eyewitness accounts, Menon also alerts us to the importance of feminist historiography. One testimony included in *No Woman's Land* is by Meghna Guhathakurta, a human-rights activist and a member of the Hindu minority in Bangladesh, who relays her mother's and grandmother's accounts of partition and Bangladesh's 1971 war of independence in order to testify to the post-partition nationalist rewriting of history. This is an urgent issue for Hindus from East Bengal who find that, as unwelcome minorities, their 'history was being systematically erased' (Menon 117).

The canon-making capacity of the anthology authorises Menon's critical response to patriarchal-nationalist discourse, a discourse that constructs women symbolically in relation to the systemic rape, abduction, and state-sponsored recovery of 'stolen women'. Feminist scholars have highlighted how partition violence targeted women as symbols of distinct communities.[11] In line with such critiques, Menon's anthology works against the narratives of nationalism, refusing to situate women as suffering victims. Instead, Menon focuses on women as active participants, who were 'involved with rebuilding lives [and who] used grit and imagination to overcome the odds—both government-induced and otherwise' (10). The anthology introduces the life narratives of women who worked as volunteers, social workers, political activists, writers, and educators during and after partition. Though Menon points out that some of them were refugees, she nonetheless stresses the agency of women working in grassroots organisations and at the level of government, who 'negotiated, subverted, manipulated or bullied, as required, to do the right thing by the women in their charge' (10).

Menon is most interested in women who crossed borders during partition, especially those working to recover women taken forcibly to live in a new community. In her analysis of the Indian government's 'Recovery Operation', she shows that the state regarded itself as the parent-protector *vis-à-vis* the enemy, Pakistan, a strategy contingent on perceiving the abducted women as passive subjects whose abductions besmirched the honour of communities. The editorial aim of *No Woman's Land* is to thwart this mythology by undermining its key presumption; accordingly the accounts in this anthology testify to an array of agency and possibilities available to women.[12] Consider, for example, the interview with Ranajit Kaur, a headmistress who returned to her pre-partition hometown in Punjab to talk with abducted and converted Sikh women. In 'Back Again, after 40 years', Kaur describes a range of responses to the experience of 'abduction'. Whereas one woman who was forcibly married protested by killing all but two of her children, others, Kaur says, did not think of themselves as 'abductees' but as women who had chosen to remain behind in their ancestral homes. According to Kaur, many women had converted and had married Sikh converts to Islam. If such marriages reinforce endogamy, they also point towards modes of resistance to the dominant Muslim group. What stands out is Kaur's assertion that, of all the women she met, she 'didn't meet a single woman there who was unhappy ... they're quite happy ... These women don't work in the fields, you see' (Menon 151). The reference to the hardships of traditional agrarian labour refuses any romantic conception of pre-partition life; in staying behind, many women eventually improved their social and economic condition.

Yet despite Kaur's attempt to uncover a latent sense of empowerment, this interview, like the other accounts in the collection, is inescapably melancholic, something Menon implicitly recognises when she states that the 'difficulty of closure [still] plagues people' (10). Melancholia functions in various forms in the testimonies of Menon's anthology. It constitutes what Khanna sees as the haunting of affect in relation to 'the weight of history', 'an epistemic violence', that continues to have palpable effects in the present (229). Manikuntala Sen's autobiographical account, 'Partition: Streams of Refugees', for instance, engages the losses of the past to demonstrate the need for political and social action. Sen's attention to the 1979 massacre of refugees on Marichjhapi in the Bengali Sundarbans identifies the *ongoing* legacies of partition. As she points out, such episodes are 'proof enough of the fact that all refugees have not been able to reach such a state of resettlement even now' (Menon 72). In a similar vein, Hasna Saha, talking of refugees in 'Trauma and Triumph', laments: 'Many are *still* adrift on either side of the border, in search of a shelter' (Menon 186, emphasis added). Here, the existence of these dispossessed and victimised groups reminds us, in Judith Butler's words, that 'the past is not past', but its material effects are very much felt in the present (472).

But just as *No Woman's Land* insists that material losses carry over into the present, it also demonstrates the persistence of psychical losses, where memories likewise encroach onto the present. In 'Two Women, One Family, Divided Nations', Sumati Guhathakurta acutely feels the loss of her son, killed during Bangladesh's war of independence, as a constant 'ache in [her] heart' (Menon 118). As she explains, '[e]ven after all these years, I feel we continue to carry the burden of Partition' (Menon 119). Similarly, for Hasna Saha, partition has both shaped and overshadowed her life. Dislocated as a child when she moved from East to West Bengal in 1948, Saha grew up in a refugee camp in Kolkata. After attending college, she returned to camp life, finding work as the general assistant of a women's refugee camp in Krishnanagar. Despite her sense of responsibility and success, Saha's comments illustrate her melancholic position, as someone who, through her experience of partition, cannot (and will not) overcome the past. Referring to her original East Bengal homeland, Saha explains:

> Bangladesh is my motherland. I can never consider it a foreign country because our language is the same, but I have no intention of visiting it, because the fond memories that I treasure of my motherland are the only possession I am left with. I do not want to lose them. (Menon 186)

The term 'motherland', in particular, invokes the contradictory meanings of Saha's exilic status as immigrant and 'Indian' national. On the one hand, it refers to Saha's identification with the modern state of Bangladesh through a common language even as Saha's refusal to visit the country symbolises a rejection of it; on the other hand, 'motherland' stands in for her childhood memories of East Bengal. These contradictions are not produced by an abstract nostalgia, but rather by the incommensurability between Saha's past and present-day Bangladesh. Saha's embrace of both positions is melancholic to the extent that it depicts her fidelity to a lost/disappeared Hindu East Bengali past ('the only possession' she has left), while allowing for her rootedness in the past (her linguistic ties to East Bengal) to reconnect her to a Muslim nation, considered separate from India. This ambivalence around identity transforms Saha's melancholic attachment into a productive course of action. It is precisely Saha's self-conscious 'introspection' into complex affiliations that resist the 'warring' mentality of exclusivist identities produced by partitioned states in a bid to ensure that history will not 'repeat itself' (Menon 186).

In *Dark Continents*, Khanna refers to a melancholia that comes out of anticolonial struggles, where '[p]olitical failures have brought about a disidentification with the nation that has failed to represent women' (230). This idea resonates within Menon's introduction to women's history during the partition of India. One specific way to contest state divisions, Menon suggests, is for women to reject *in toto* the notion of nationhood. Because the nation is an 'intrinsically male' construct, Menon sees it as circumscribing and excluding women; an understanding reflected through her anthology's title *No Woman's Land* and confirmed by her conversations with women about partition (4). As she explains:

> women were bartered like oranges and apples; apportioned between countries according to official classification—Hindu, Muslim, Sikh; minor; legitimate or illegitimate; abducted or not; forcibly converted vs. voluntarily married—with no choice or rights in the matter. Not only do women have no country, they cannot even call their bodies their own . . . .
>
> Years later, in the course of our research, when we met widows and destituted [sic] women at the Karnal Mahila Ashram in Haryana (India), they still spoke of Mianwali or Montgomery or Abbottabad or Sagodha or Multan or Sialkot as home. 'Now there is no country', said Somavanti to us. 'This is not ours, that is no longer ours.' (Menon 7–8)

Melancholia functions as part of a feminist practice that responds to the injustices perpetrated by the nation-state. In this feminist melancholia, we see the beginnings of a politics that holds onto the losses of the past and allows for what Menon sees as women's transnational affiliations across partitioned states.

A further aspect of melancholia that relates to the failures of the state can be identified in the autobiographical accounts of Kambalen Patel.[13] As a social worker, Patel was actively involved in the Indian government's recovery work of abducted women after partition; her autobiography describes some of the recovery cases through Special Tribunals set up by the Indian and Pakistani governments. Given a central position in *No Woman's Land* (three excerpts of her autobiography are included), Patel narrates how her life has been shaped by her involvement in recovering children and women from Pakistan. Through these encounters, Patel, like Butalia, bears witness to the suffering during partition and testifies to the enduring and unsettling instances of emotions that haunt her. Alongside this haunting, Patel divulges a sense of loss that suggests what Khanna has called a 'melancholic recognition of the suffering of another as one's own "unjustifiable violation"' (230). This stems in particular from the tension between Patel's experiences as a social worker and the (unknowable) repercussions of this work in people's lives. A conscientious worker, Patel is proud of both her work and her empathic ties to the people in her charge; simultaneously, she condemns the government's emotional detachment from the lives it repatriates and questions the legitimacy of such work. Detailing her feelings of sorrow, despair, guilt, anger, and the 'terrible strain' of her work (Menon 162), Patel's testimony distances this autobiographical subject from the cold logic and formalism of governmental institutions. Yet, such emotions also serve to remind us of Patel's complicity within the state. We can see Patel's autobiography as a mode of questioning of governmental involvement that also asks for the reader's sympathy for her own conflicted position of circumscribed agency. She represents the government, carrying out governmental work even as she is criticised by other workers for being 'swept away by emotion' (Menon 170); but she is also powerfully caught up in the lives of the people she repatriates and acutely feels 'one blow after another' as the recovery process, frequently operating beyond her control, damages multiple lives (Menon 162). Patel's melancholia comes out of a lack of closure as well as her empathy for partition's victims. In recalling her memories of the past and other people's 'misery and suffering' (Menon 175), Patel is left to struggle with a sense of culpability and sorrow.

In the excerpt from her autobiography, entitled 'Lock up your Heart', Patel reflects on the importance of emotions, which, as elsewhere in the anthology, call the reader for an empathic emotional response as a way to overcome communal divides. At the beginning of her narrative, Patel describes being escorted by a police officer who points out a well where Sikh women had committed suicide. As the officer laments, we 'have not been able to protect the women of our own locality ... [we] abduct[ed] the mothers and sisters of our fellow human beings', Patel notes that his eyes are filling with tears (Menon 166). She is surprised to discover that he is not a refugee, but is, in fact, a local who had not sustained any losses during partition, and who had helped a number of Hindu friends leave safely. The officer's account communicates his suffering through feelings of collective guilt ('How sternly will posterity judge us?'); but at an individual level, he bears the cost of his community's actions, finding that he is lonely and isolated without his Hindu friends despite 'living in the midst of [his] own community' (Menon 167). For Patel, the man's emotion haunts her, his 'agony ... stayed with me for a long time', evidence of the harm perpetrated by partition in unravelling complex multireligious communities (Menon 167).

A similar melancholia can be identified in Patel's other excerpts in Menon's anthology, 'Ismat and Jatin' and 'Abandoned', where the haunting of affects relates to a sense of failure, guilt, and anguish. Forced by the government to repatriate an unwilling woman, Ismat, to her parents in Pakistan, Patel feels partly responsible when Ismat's cross-communal marriage to a Hindu, Jatin, disintegrates. Once home, Ismat had succumbed to family pressure, 'transformed' utterly, and denounced her husband, refusing to ever see him again

(Menon 162). This incident is a shock to Patel, breaking with Jatin's trust, (as well as Patel's belief) in her social work. As she writes, the experience 'had so shaken my entire being that even as I write these lines today, I feel I have not been able to recover from it completely' (Menon 162). As with the officer's 'agony', what can be traced here is a melancholic awareness of collective guilt and communal failures. In both cases, the traumatic experience of broken families and communities carries within it a melancholic residue that circulates between people and continues to upset Patel many years later. 'Abandoned' also exemplifies a portrait of this melancholia as Patel struggles to confront her involvement with separated families.

'Abandoned', as the title suggests, encapsulates the harsh and melancholy fate of illegitimate babies, born as a result of abductions and forced marriages during partition. The recovered women were allowed to keep their children, but this incurred a serious problem when relatives came for them, since a 'child born to a Hindu mother by a Muslim father was hardly acceptable' (Menon 177). Many of the women kept their children a secret, and eventually had to abandon them in order to return to their families. Patel writes of the difficulty of this situation and her inability to retain responsibility to the mothers and their children:

> We had made a number of promises to their mothers at the time of parting about how we would personally look after them, but these proved false as we ourselves could not see them again. Even today when I remember their mothers sobbing, my heart aches with sorrow. (Menon 179)

Patel's recurring and painful memories of 'sobbing' bear witness to her melancholia, suggesting not only a level of vicarious trauma but, again, calling attention to feelings of guilt. In delineating the melancholia of these partition accounts, I see not a pessimistic view of haunting, but rather an ongoing engagement with lingering traumatic affects that articulate political disillusionment with national narratives. As Patel's account indicates, melancholia conveys an awareness of partition's legacies that are supposedly in the distant past. In many ways, such melancholia reminds us, in the words of Eng and Kazanjian, that 'the past remains steadfastly alive in the present' (4).

The affective power of this melancholia, conveyed by the different voices and recollections of women, reminds the reader that, in the wake of partition, if there is no healing or reconciliation, there are still available modes of (re)action, of resisting partitionist divides, and engaging with the past. The production of partition anthologies precipitates a new politics of being in the world. As anthologies circulate within the educational spheres of India and other Anglophonic countries, they carry those traumatic affects and so these pedagogical tools function to institutionalise and testify to the extent of partition's traumatic history. The role of such work is particularly significant if we consider the growing output of partition scholarship by the South Asian intelligentsia. The work produced by academics, such as Butalia and the editors of the partition anthologies, repositions partition as a central concern in academic scholarship and, by extension, within public discourse. Indeed, the growing body of partition work in South Asia demonstrates the power of affective charges, since earlier work clearly spurs the intelligentsia to both reproduce and cultivate their own comparative enquiries. These models of partition scholarship not only speak to the ways in which the partition subject is profoundly shaped by the trauma and the affects of the past, but also offer fruitful ground for the public recognition of partition's traumas and for the emergence of new forms of moral responsibility.

Notes

[1] The discourse surrounding partition, as in Holocaust studies, often signifies the importance of the event by use of a capital letter. However, Jill Didur makes a strong argument for using a lower-case 'p' precisely in order to avoid 'monumentaliz[ing] the events in question' (165 n2).

[2] For more details on anthologies and their pedagogical implications, see Jeffrey Di Leo (esp. 60–84).

[3] For an exception to this, see Jasodhara Bagchi and Subhoranjan Dasgupta.

[4] Peritext must be understood as distinct from paratext. The latter conceives of editorial apparatuses as distinct from and, in some ways, supplementary to the primary texts, the literary texts. By peritext, I refer to the governing editorial spirit that manages the production of the entire anthology. A peritext should be understood as that which encloses and suffuses the entire work. A peritext thus has as much to contribute to our understanding of an introduction, headnotes, or footnotes, as it does to selective criteria.

[5] Though the word communal usually applies to communities and communitarian forms of belonging, in the context of Indian history, the term designates religious communities.

[6] The point here is not to disregard the work of Mikhail Bakhtin by suggesting that novels are single-voiced texts, whose ability to represent partition is subordinate to the heteroglossic anthology. Merely, the fact remains that the contributions to an anthology are, at the very least, produced independently of a supervening author and as such can reasonably be expected to function in a different type of antagonism than the multiple voices held in tension by the novelistic genre.

[7] Intellectuals have played a prominent part in the public construction of collective trauma in various contexts, such as the commemoration of the Holocaust and African American trauma of slavery. Frequently the bearers of social capital and endowed with institutional authority, academics have long had an important role in the public sphere for advancing claims. See Jeffrey C. Alexander et al. (esp. 60–111).

[8] In Bangla, the language of Bengal, Bangladesh refers to the country of Bengal. This term, like the poem, pre-dates the formation of the political state of Bangladesh.

[9] See Sengupta (ii).

[10] Menon can be faulted for her assumption that a 'gendered perspective' entails only female accounts. As Priyamvada Gopal has brilliantly demonstrated, partition also led to 'ensuing crises of [the] male self and sexuality' (90). Though this article does not focus on the intricacies of Menon's feminist analysis, some of her claims need to be critiqued. For instance, her overtures to an implicitly shared womanhood risks essentialising and homogenising different subjectivities. This can be further traced in her emphasis on women's ability to act and demand change; Menon's examples of

such female agency are, in fact, predicated upon the socio-economic privileges of class and education. Menon's focus on women as agents also leaves aside the role of women as perpetrators of violence, though the autobiographies she includes call attention to this fact. See Menon (62).

[11] See Urvashi Butalia; Veena Das; Jill Didur; Sangeeta Ray.

[12] Menon and Bhasin also make this point in *Borders and Boundaries* (91).

[13] Patel's testimony also features in Menon and Bhasin's *Borders and Boundaries*, though the experiences she relates are different. There she also talks about her experience working for the Indian Government's Recovery Operation of abducted women in Pakistan. But her focus is more on the dilemmas of the abductees and offering a general overview of her experiences, rather than delving at length into specific cases and into her own feelings of personal and emotional involvement.

References

Ahmed, Sara. *The Cultural Politics of Emotion*. Edinburgh: Edinburgh UP, 2004.

Alexander, Jeffrey C., Ron Eyerman, Bernard Giesen, Neil J. Smelser, and Piotr Sztompka. *Cultural Trauma and Collective Identity*. Berkeley: U of California P, 2004.

Bagchi, Jasodhara, and Subhoranjan Dasgupta, eds. *The Trauma and the Triumph: Gender and Partition in Eastern India*. Kolkata: Stree, 2003.

Bhalla, Alok. *Stories about the Partition of India*. 3 vols. New Delhi: HarperCollins, 1994.

Butalia, Urvashi. *The Other Side of Silence: Voices From the Partition of India*. 1999. Durham: Duke University Press, 2000.

Butler, Judith. 'Afterword: After Loss, What Then?' *Loss: The Politics of Mourning*. Ed. David Eng and David Kazanjian. Berkeley: U of California P, 2003. 467–73.

Cleary, Joe. *Literature, Partition and the Nation-State: Culture and Conflict in Ireland, Israel, and Palestine*. Cambridge: Cambridge UP, 2002.

Das, Veena. 'The Act of Witnessing: Violence, Poisonous Knowledge, and Subjectivity.' *Violence and Subjectivity*. Ed. Veena Das et al. Berkeley: U of California P, 2000. 205–25.

Didur, Jill. *Unsettling Partition: Literature, Gender, Memory*. Toronto: U of Toronto P, 2006.

Di Leo, Jeffrey, ed. *On Anthologies: Politics and Pedagogy*. Lincoln: U of Nebraska P, 2004.

Eng, David, and David Kazanjian, eds. *Loss: The Politics of Mourning*. Berkeley: U of California P, 2003.

Freud, Sigmund. 'Mourning and Melancholia.' 1915. *The Standard Edition of the Complete Psychological Works of Sigmund Freud*. Ed. James Strachey. Vol. 14. London: Vintage, 2001. 243–58.

Gopal, Priyamvada. *Literary Radicalism in India: Gender, Nation, and the Transition to Independence*. New York: Routledge, 2005.

Hirsch, Marianne. Family Frames: Photography, Narrative, and Postmemory. Cambridge, MA: Harvard UP, 1997.

——. 'Surviving Images: Holocaust Photographs and the Work of Postmemory.' *The Yale Journal of Criticism* 14.1 (2001): 5–37.

Kabir, Ananya Jahanara. 'Gender, Memory, Trauma: Women's Novels on the Partition of India.' *Comparative Studies of South Asia, Africa, and the Middle-East* 25.1 (2005): 177–90.

Kamboureli, Smaro. *Scandalous Bodies: Diasporic Literature in English Canada*. Don Mills, ON: Oxford UP, 2000.

Khanna, Ranjana. *Dark Continents: Psychoanalysis and Colonialism*. Durham: Duke UP, 2003.

LaCapra, Dominick. *Writing History, Writing Trauma*. Baltimore: Johns Hopkins UP, 2001.

Menon, Ritu, ed. *No Woman's Land: Women from Pakistan, India, and Bangladesh Write on the Partition of India*. New Delhi: Women Unlimited, 2004.

Menon, Ritu, and Kamla Bhasin. *Borders and Boundaries: Women in India's Partition*. New Brunswick, NJ: Rutgers UP, 1998.

Nandy, Ashis. 'The Days of the Hyaena: A Foreword.' *Mapmaking: Partition Stories from 2 Bengals*. ed. Debjani Sengupta. New Delhi: Srishti, 2003. i–xi.

Ray, Sangeeta. *En-gendering India: Woman and Nation in Colonial and Postcolonial Narratives*. Durham: Duke UP, 2000.

Santner, Eric L. *On Creaturely Life: Rilke, Benjamin, Sebald*. Chicago: U of Chicago P, 2006.

Schaffer, Kay, and Sidonie Smith. *Human Rights and Narrated Lives: The Ethics of Recognition*. New York: Palgrave MacMillan, 2004.

Sengupta, Debjani, ed. *Mapmaking: Partition Stories from 2 Bengals*. New Delhi: Srishti, 2003.

Thrift, Nigel. 'Intensities of Feeling: Towards a Spatial Politics of Affect.' *Geografiska Annaler Series* B.86 (2004): 57–78.

'I Must Know': Re-membering Native Women in the CAVNET_IW Community

Jane Haladay

Historical and Media Violence toward Native North American Women

Despite the dramatic expansion of digital communications technologies and the interest in trauma narratives over the past several decades, representing the traumatic life stories of specific populations—including the exorbitant level of violence against Native North American women—remains a small tributary in the larger current of mainstream news. In both the United States and Canada, the disproportionate rate of sexual violence against Native/American Indian, Alaska Native, and First Nations women is consistently underreported, illustrating the contention of anthropologist Kyra Landzelius that 'journalism is biased *tout court* and at the outset, biased in prioritizing (or conversely erasing) some issues over others; biased in following, writing and posting certain stories in lieu of alternatives,' despite the potential for more expansive and equitable coverage in online journalism (28). Indeed, as Amnesty International concluded in April 2007, despite centuries of brutalisation of Indigenous women under colonial regimes, of the 'many incidents of sexual violence against American Indian and Alaska native women [...] the great majority of stories remain[s] untold' (*Maze of Injustice* 4).

For various and intricate reasons, many Indigenous women choose not to tell their stories, both within and beyond their home communities. Because sexual violence directed at Native women has been used in the so-called 'Americas' as a tool of colonial genocide and resource control for the past five centuries, and because 'race' and gender cannot be separated when considering violence against women of colour, scholar Andrea Smith declares that 'Communities of color ... often advocate that women keep silent about sexual and domestic violence in order to maintain a united front against racism' (1). As Native women are particularly aware, a 'united front' continues to be necessary to combat the dysfunctional, racist U.S. legal system that has 'created a complex interrelation between ... [tribal, state, and federal] jurisdictions that undermines equality before the law and often allows perpetrators to evade justice. In some cases this has created areas of effective lawlessness which encourages violence' (*Maze of Injustice* 8).

Several signification pieces of legislation have worked in combination over time to create the 'effective lawlessness' affecting Native women on Tribal lands.[1] Perhaps the most insidious is the 1978 Supreme Court Case Oliphant v. Suquamish Indian Tribe, which divests Tribal authorities of the power to prosecute non-Natives who commit crimes on Native lands. Legal analyst Sarah Deer explains that the Oliphant decision:

> has created a crisis situation in some tribal communities, because non-Indian sexual predators, drug manufacturers, pimps, and other violent persons have become attracted to Indian country as a location in which crimes can be committed without recourse (Fletcher, 2004). Indian country has become attractive to pedophiles and sexual predators, because of the vulnerability of the citizens and jurisdictional gaps. (22)

Historically preceding *Oliphant* is the Major Crimes Act (MCA) of 1885, which has allowed for the federal prosecution of felonies, including rape and murder, committed on Tribal lands. Most Tribes have widely interpreted the MCA to require federal prosecution of felonies, although in fact Tribes may prosecute these cases themselves. Once felony cases are referred to federal authorities, they enter a system notorious for its protracted and indifferent response to administering justice to female and child victims of violence. Thus, notes Deer, '[m]any tribes do not pursue cases against rapists and batterers, or will wait until a declination from a federal or state prosecutor before proceeding with an official tribal response' ('Federal Indian Law' 20). These jurisdictional tangles on Tribal lands have led to large majority (up to 86% of reported cases) of sexual abuse against Native women being perpetrated by non-Native men, a circumstance that is unique compared to other ethnic and so-called 'racial' groups in the United States (*Maze of Injustice* 4-5).

Clearly, as Deer observes, through its consistent erosion of Native sovereignty over time, 'The laws and policies of the United States play a significant role in the high rate of victimization, because they have inhibited the ability of Tribal communities to respond to and address crime in a culturally appropriate way' ('Federal Indian Law' 19). In this rigged context of ongoing colonial oppression and aggression, violence against Native women has become normalised, and many women view living in a state of trauma as inevitable. Deer emphasises that, 'Criminal victimization and trauma has a profound impact on the future of indigenous nations. Without an adequate system for resolution and healing,' she adds, 'psychological trauma and victimization create a cyclical sense of despair and desperation, indeed, a very continuation of the colonization process' ('Federal Indian Law' 25). Because the forces of colonisation continue to impact Native peoples, living with trauma becomes a historical legacy that is often transmitted to future generations, as health professionals Bonnie Duran, Eduardo Duran, and Maria Yellow Horse Brave Heart explain:

> Historical trauma and its effects are complex, multigenerational, and cumulative. A constellation of features that occur in reaction to multigenerational, collective, historical, and cumulative psychic wounding over time—over the lifespan and across generations—historical trauma is characterized as incomplete mourning and the resulting depression absorbed by children from birth onward. Unresolved trauma is intergenerationally cumulative, thus compounding the mental health problems of succeeding generations. (64)

While Amnesty's 113-page report goes far in painting a broader, more contextualised portrait of the root causes and contemporary circumstances of violence against Native women in the United States, more common daily news coverage—when it occurs at all—typically takes the form of truncated narratives outlining minimal facts around women's violent experiences; often, these include graphic details about a woman's torture and death. Mainstream media narratives of the specific stories of women victimised by violence serve at once to report on the unvarnished facts of their violent victimisation and, potentially, to reinscribe trauma for women who read these fractured, disturbing narratives about the lives and deaths of their relatives and friends. Whether intentionally or not, these mainstream representations perpetuate a form of narrative violence against Native women by only rarely and partially representing the complexities of their lives. As a result, 'The extent to which Native peoples are not seen as 'real' people in the larger colonial discourse,' observes Andrea Smith, 'indicates the success of sexual violence, among other racist and colonialist forces, in destroying the perceived humanity of Native peoples' (12).

Resistance and Truth-Telling through CAVNET_IW

Concurrent with past and present histories of colonially based violence against Native women are, of course, the resistance efforts of Native women themselves. Generations of Indigenous women have long been asserting their own stories around the trauma of violence against them and their relatives, communities, and homelands in ways that work toward making whole what colonialism attempts to systematically dismember. One particularly powerful contemporary venue of re-membering the piecemeal and partial representations of violence against Native women in mainstream U.S. news is the U.S.-based internet community CAVNET_IW (Communities Against Violence Network—Indigenous Women), whose formation, intentions, and practices serve as a potent counter-narrative to the mainstream news media's consistent efforts to render Native women's stories invisible and insignificant. As a site that not only disseminates news about violence against Indigenous women but creates a forum for women to tell their own stories, CAVNET_IW has fashioned a potential safe space through which immediate and historical trauma affecting Native women paves pathways to personal healing and political change. As scholars Kay Schaffer and Sidonie Smith have noted, 'new media technologies extend the scope for the production of testimony, sustaining new social movements and styles of political activism. They engage victims on the local level in ways that help to destabilize state power and build transformative transnational alliances, albeit in uneven, contingent, and unpredictable ways' (39). Through its digital community—whose 'homeland' is virtual rather than geographic—CAVNET_IW generates discourses around trauma that are fluid, multi-layered, and develop through list members' long-term participation over time.

At the same time CAVNET_IW offers a virtual sanctuary for members working with issues of Indigenous women's violence, it also grapples with the slippery unpredictability of the myriad complexities of virtual all-text discourse. These include the impossibility of discerning tone and accessing facial expressions, body language, and those other communicative markers of face-to-face, real-time human interaction that are also integral to Indigenous oral traditions, with the result that '[s]ome stories, formerly locked in silence, open wounds and re-trigger traumatic feelings once they are told' (Schaffer and Smith 4). Thus, while 'the contexts of story production, circulation, and reception' (Schaffer and Smith 5) created on CAVNET_IW serve as a powerful mode of resistance to colonial culture's silencing of Native women's traumatic experiences through maintaining the circulation of narratives necessary to forge activism, the impact of these traumatic narratives even upon list members cannot ultimately be controlled. Paradoxically, then, the work of CAVNET_IW to end violence and heal trauma is partly enacted through keeping episodes of traumatic violence constantly present in the consciousness of list members through the circulation and witnessing of life stories. CAVNET_IW is also a space where members reflect upon and attempt to work through the ethical issues raised by this production and reception of trauma story online.

CAVNET_IW is a carefully monitored discussion space requiring member subscription and message screening before posting. While CAVNET_IW makes no claims to represent a specific Indigenous cultural community, or even a 'pan-Native' community (CAVNET_IW is also peopled by non-Native subscribers, and by both men and women), and while its primary language is English, CAVNET_IW's activist methods of re-circulating and deconstructing traumatic narratives enacts traditional Indigenous cultural practices of transmitting cultural and historical knowledges through continuing to tell the stories of the people, no matter how painful, as a form of education, remembrance, and survival. CAVNET_IW re-members and re-embodies Native women by disseminating a consistent and multidimensional stream of information in a forum 'in which issues facing Native women [are] paramount' (Deer 'My responses').

Deer, Victim Advocacy Legal Specialist for the Tribal Law & Policy Institute in Saint Paul, Minnesota, and a citizen of the Mvskoke (Creek) Nation, has 'co-moderated'[2] CAVNET-IW in a private capacity since the group's inception on August 31, 2001; currently, she is its primary moderator. Deer explains that 'This listserv started in 2001 and my hope was always that it would be a discussion-based list. It has kind of morphed over time into a news service, with occasional discussion' (Message #4173).[3] Because list members participate in contextualising partial mass media representations of Native women affected by violence, and because of the multiplicity of women's narratives of personal and collective trauma and resistance represented by CAVNET_IW, the group helps subvert static and stereotypical representations of Native women and their communities. Internet user groups like CAVNET_IW offer powerful opportunities to destabilise and talk back to dominant power regimes and are especially significant, as Landzelius observes, 'for indigenous peoples, who have long been de-legitimized by ruling cultural norms and isolated (economically, politically, geographically) from centers of influence' (1).

In terms of mainstream media critique, Deer states that, 'I am always especially heartened when Native advocates post a response to an article which is racist or otherwise missing an important point. I like to see the 'real world' critique of the way the media portrays us' ('My responses'). She notes that while she would like to see many more responses to posts by CAVNET_IW list participants, she is sensitive to the cultural factors that may influence some members' willingness and/or comfort level with publicly posting comments to the list:

> I think Native people, particularly those who are more traditional, are hesitant to put their story 'out there' into cyberspace where it may be forwarded or used in

> other contexts. I have heard that sometimes people want to post, but they aren't sure how or are worried about losing control over their story. ('My responses')

This very legitimate fear of losing control over personal and/or community representation results from the ongoing theft and misrepresentation of Aboriginal and Native voice, stories, and other cultural property by colonising institutions and individuals, including the mainstream media, that have traumatised Native peoples for centuries. Schaffer and Smith emphasise this point in relation to colonial assumptions about Indigenous people's willingness to tell their personal stories in colonial public venues related to human rights reparations. They posit that:

> when personal stories are transformed into testimony ... for an official inquiry.... [colonial institutions] operate on the assumption that people, when given the occasion, will and should want to tell their stories. This presumption occludes the cultural rights of potential witnesses who may need to protect themselves, their community, their history, and their secret knowledges by remaining silent. (40)

Respecting these people's concerns, Deer envisions future developments that will allow members to post anonymously, and so share stories of trauma, healing, encouragement, or advice without revealing their individual identities unless they choose to do so.

Deer first became involved with the larger CAVNET list late in 2000 while working at the Department of Justice, where she met Marc Dubin, Esq., former Special Counsel to the Office on Violence Against Women at the Justice Department and Executive Director of CAVNET.[4] Deer expressed to Dubin her belief in 'the need to have a separate forum for Native women's issues' in light of 'the way in which [she'd] seen Native women's issues marginalized in [the] larger discourse about violence against women' ('My responses'). Because similar feelings of hopelessness, isolation, and despair affecting Native women victimised by violence can also affect those women and men who work on their behalf, cultivating a climate of solidarity and supportive community is the first of CAVNET_IW's five primary goals. Deer founded CAVNET_IW, a Yahoo! Group, to 'Stay in touch with other advocates and professionals working in Indian country and/or with Indigenous women' in order to '[w]ork against the isolation that is so prevalent in our work,' and to '[s]hare ideas and resources on how to help empower Indigenous women who are victimized by violence' (CAVNET_IW). Beyond providing concrete announcements and information about conferences, trainings, legislation, and breaking news, CAVNET_IW strives to explore 'ways that services and advocacy for women survivors can be designed to address the cultural and spiritual needs of Indigenous women' (CAVNET_IW).

Since its inception in 2001 until November 26, 2008 (the date of this writing), CAVNET_IW has posted a total of 5,664 messages to a membership of 304 subscribers (CAVNET_IW). CAVNET_IW provides such practical items as phone numbers for safe houses, job opportunities, and dates for trainings and survivor workshops alongside spiritual, psychological, and emotional support in the form of member posts, posts on legislative or community successes in anti-violence work, and even an occasional inspirational poem, such as Audre Lorde's 'A Litany for Survival' ('Poem,' Message #126). Not all information on the list outlines traumatic material, yet each post is related to aspects of violence against Native women and anti-violence activism. 'Beginning in 2001 when CAVNET_IW started, every article is saved and searchable,' says Deer. 'Therefore, I have been contacted by numerous academics, students, and activists about using the archives for their work. There is simply no other such database of articles available about Native women anywhere in the world' ('My responses').

Bearing the Weight of Traumatic Remembrance

To witness and digitally re-member through language (CAVNET_IW distributes only text-based messages) the lives of Native women affected by violence is ceaseless, often painful labour for anti-violence workers, survivors, and their friends, relatives, and communities. Making space to re-embody Indigenous women within the multiplicity of CAVNET_IW's digital archives and email posts can be simultaneously exhilarating and exhausting for the list community, and for Deer as the list's primary moderator. The volume of information detailing graphic violence against Native women can be traumatic in part because this violence is at once a constant feature of contemporary Native experience and a subject that remains chronically absent from regular mainstream news coverage as part of continuing colonial efforts at Indigenous erasure. Through CAVNET_IW, 'Survivor narratives tell stories of abuse through which narrators turn themselves from victims to survivors through acts of speaking out that shift attention to systemic causes of violation' (Schaffer and Smith 28). Thus, the nurturing of digital communities such as CAVNET_IW is essential in anti-violence efforts for Native women, since stories of affirmation, hope, anti-violence victories, and Indigenous self-determination share space with the stream of traumatic narratives.

In moderating CAVNET_IW, Deer confesses she has 'often expressed the worry that CAVNET_IW is 'too depressing,'' and fears that her 'constant posting of news articles about Native women who have been beaten, raped, murdered, or gone missing makes the nature of the listserv simply too demoralizing and depressing.' However, in communicating virtually and in person with list members, she often finds that members appreciate the posting of traumatic stories. These members tell Deer that:

> for so long our stories (Native women's stories) of being victimized have been invisibilized. While we can turn on network television and hear the stories of countless murdered and missing White women – there is very little discussion about the high rates of violence experienced by Native women. The CAVNET_IW listserv, by publicizing and highlighting our stories into a larger forum, it creates a

> sense of community around the stories. Subscribers have mentioned offering prayers and ceremony for women they read about on CAVNET_IW. ('My responses')

List members understand that the purpose of CAVNET_IW is to keep visible the stories of Indigenous women affected by violence; still, it is inevitable that Deer's concerns over posting traumatic narratives that negatively impact list members are occasionally realised. CAVNET_IW list members—many of whom are violence survivors themselves—are at different points in their journeys of remembrance, testimony, and healing. One brief news item Deer posted on April 5, 2007, serves as a potent example. While there are frequently animated exchanges critiquing and discussing specific information that is posted to the group, this article precipitated a particularly emotional exchange that demonstrates Schaffer and Smith's contention that once stories of suffering reach broader audiences through mass reproduction, 'those audiences subject the narrative to different and unpredictable readings' (32). Further, through public testimony and/or documentation, 'stories can be subjected to further scrutiny and response, including acceptance and recognition but also challenge, rebuttal, scorn, and denial' (44).

The emotional, conflicting ways in which the original traumatic news narrative about the death of Marisol Padilla was received and deployed by CAVNET_IW list members underscores the reality that narrative reception cannot be predicted or policed, perhaps especially—though certainly not exclusively—in virtual media, where narrative replication takes place instantaneously and abundantly. The story describing Padilla's death, posted under the subject heading 'Woman Found Dead On Reservation Identified,' was (relative to other narratives posted on the CAVNET_IW list) short, with a minimum of graphic, though disturbing, details. The article did not identify whether Padilla herself is a Native woman. Following is the entire article as posted:

> A woman found Saturday shot in the arm and hanged, naked, from a tree on the Tohono O'Odham Indian Reservation has been identified.
> Marisol Padilla, 32, was a Tucson resident and not from the reservation. Not much else is known about her at this time.
> Padilla's body was discovered around noon over the weekend near milepost 15 on South Mission Road, when Pima County Sheriff's officers responded to a call from a passerby.
>
> Although Padilla was shot in the arm, the wound was not fatal. Investigators are waiting for autopsy results to determine the cause of death.
> (Marissa Pasquet, Message #4146)

Five days after this item was posted, a list member, 'Diana,' re-sent this news article with a brief prefacing note stating, 'This woman was terrorized and tortured before she was killed.'[5] It was apparently this brief postscript, and not the original graphic details in the article about Padilla's death, that incited the impassioned response of a fellow list member, 'Lauren,' who immediately posted the following:

> what is the purpose of this note? it is obvious that this woman suffered greatly. i often question the purpose of sending these types of notes around to all. ours is a world where this behavior occurs. we know this reality. what good is brought about by highlighting these instances of depravity? it is likely that those on this listserv are already too familiar with this type of violence. i think it does no good to spread this around. if there is a need to 'spread' this news around, it should be to the non-Indian, non-academic, non-activist population whom might benefit from knowing this behavior continues to occur. i would imagine that, like myself, those who subscribe to this listserv are disserviced and, perhaps, unnecessarily jolted and even traumatized when they open their email to this type of revelation. i would ask that some type of warning be made to tell the reader that the note being circulated contains disturbing content so that the reader will be able to decide if she/he wants/needs/should be subjected to this type of news. i HATE waking up to my e-mail that contains these types of messages when I haven't even had the opportunity to decide if this is they type of material with which I want to start my day. thank you. (Message #4167)

Only hours after the original post, and before the string of responses evoked by Lauren's message began to be posted that same day, Lauren unsubscribed from CAVNET_IW.

Lauren's message points to the dual reality that CAVNET_IW list members are both acutely aware of the narratives of violence circulated through the list, yet they still may be 'simultaneously jolted and even traumatized' to read these stories. Because of the nature of information disseminated through CAVNET_IW, the list is never neutral or easily definable terrain. The ensuing conversation elicited by Lauren's message raises several significant themes: that traumatic narratives are part and parcel of the work CAVNET_IW is committed to witnessing through recirculation and archiving; that these narratives will consistently evoke various and powerful responses from list members who read them; and, that it is up to individual members to find ways to regulate their consumption of traumatic narratives to maintain their own emotional, physical, psychic, and spiritual health.

First to respond to Lauren's message was Diana. Her remarks, while lengthy, I reproduce here in their entirety because they provide cogent analysis of the stresses of working on a daily basis with traumatised individuals and communities, while attempting to utilise a virtual community like CAVNET_IW to consistently balance truth-telling and the witnessing of traumatic experience with respectful, ethical self-expression. Further, Diana's analysis of the original news story's representation of violence against women, both in what it does and does not state, focuses attention on several of the major issues—including non-Native perpetrators' conscious exploitation of Native lands to commit violent crimes against Native women—that CAVNET_IW list members are dedicated to exposing and resisting:

> Hey, listen, [Lauren] . . I make no apology for my note. I've been in this business a long time and find that lots of times people have their own issues that they are working on resolving which cause them to react in a particularly strong way to certain material. However, in my humble opinion, that doesn't mean that I have to walk around on eggshells and while I am respectful and professional with others in my daily walk through life I cannot take the blame for someone else's reaction when the nature of the internet is that there is lots of information that is sent out there to anonymous folks (on a listserv in this case) and there is some level of self-selected participation in it. I suggest that if you have found you would prefer not to read CAVNET_IW emails or reactions to them that you either unsubscribe or hit the delete button before reading. There are other ways to deal with your reactions than attacking a fellow listserv member who happened to post a comment.
>
> I don't think I have to justify my comments or reaction to a particular news story. Is there some rule heretofore unbeknownst to me which states that listserv members cannot post their reactions or observations to an article? In fact, I wish that we had more reaction and interaction on this listserv (it seems to me there is a tendency to day-after-day read the vast number of articles of victimization with no listserv reaction whatsoever which seems more of a disservice from my perspective). The news article struck me as particularly demonstrative of violence against women that includes clear elements of torture and actual victim terrorization prior to carrying out a premeditated murder. It is somewhat qualitatively different than some of the other information we receive over this listserv in my view because it points to a particular kind of offender who then dumps his victim on a reservation in Indian Country (the article said that this victim was not from the reservation). This has enormous implications not only for victims of violence but for Indian Country as well. This is some of the good that comes from commenting. And, we might even have some kind of reaction discussion to the material we receive on this listserv. Why shouldn't I comment even at the risk of others being 'jolted'? What is it about my comment that is unusually jolting or traumatizing, especially given that you admit that you already knew that the torture element existed simply by reading the article?
>
> Everyone makes a choice to sustain a risk of exposure to unwanted material by opening their email everyday. I can't prevent that or protect you from that ... or is it your suggestion that we should all just read the articles and delete?
>
> I just don't get your protest ... and I don't even think it's legitimate. I don't think it's helpful for you to attack me for attempting to contribute to some sort of discussion on this listserv! (Message #4170)

Diana's articulation of individual group members' 'risk of exposure to unwanted material' by opening the emails disseminated via the CAVNET_IW list ironically underscores the core problematic of circulating traumatic narratives to list members in the first place. As a dual site of information dissemination and the public voicing of traumatic episodes involving violence against Native women, trauma is simultaneously named, witnessed, and/or reanimated, depending on the personal circumstances of individual member reception at the time of her reading a specific story. Still, the responses of the approximately ten list members who participated in this thread underscore that traumatic stories do need to be told, despite the periodically overwhelming pain elicited by regularly reading a superabundance of tales focusing on brutality and loss. Several members who responded remarked that although for various reasons they 'rarely comment on the listserv' (Vicki Ybanez, Message #4171) or 'rarely engage in the discussion process over this venue' (Tawna Sanchez, Message #4172)—a fact that Diana also critiques in her message above—they are extraordinarily appreciative of CAVNET_IW as a forum for circulating what might otherwise become the lost or silenced stories of their violated sisters, mothers, daughters, and friends.

For most members, Deer's posting of traumatic events and narratives on CAVNET_IW is part of the imperative community building and informational outreach process that compels survivors, anti-violence advocates, and other list members to join CAVNET_IW. 'I personally find it [CAVNET_IW] to be helpful as we all run the risk of isolating or insulating ourselves,' noted Tawna Sanchez, Family Services Director of the Native American Youth and Family Center, in her April 12 message:

> Reading all of your views and concerns regarding various issues has been helpful in many ways and it is good to know that I am not alone in my views. As service providers in one way or another we all run the risk of vicarious trauma just because of what we do and who we are in our communities. However, if I know what has happened in another part of Indian country I can better address more local issues as not an isolated incident, because we know they are not. Another woman has lost her life to violence and that should be recognized as such. It should also be recognized that where her body was found could have a significant backlash on Native people wherever they are. We cannot ignore either of these issues because they do affect our communities. I may not always be ready for all the gory details of a case like this, but I do need to know what is happening in order to better protect my own community. (Message #4172)

'I, too, am one of the silent readers of this listserv,' wrote Nicole Gray, Public Outreach Coordinator for the Montana Coalition Against Domestic & Sexual Violence (MCADSV). 'I echo what others have said: there are times when the e-mails are hard emotionally to read. But it's important to me that I read what I can. It drives home, for me, the need to be an active part of the movement for social change and justice.' (Message #4184)

At this point in the thread, Deer posted a message as CAVNET_IW moderator, outlining her choices and philosophy in posting specific information to the list. 'Certainly my intent is not to trigger/traumatize any readers,' Deer explained:

> [...] My motivations in posting news stories about horrible things that happen to us is that we need to hold the systems accountable. It is hard to hold the systems accountable if we don't know what is happening. I know these news stories are just the tip of the iceberg. Usually when something happens to Native women, reporters don't bother to cover it. I find the few stories out there and try to share them with you all in an effort to stay informed (Message #4173).

Deer's remarks underscore her goal to see CAVENT_IW continue to further develop into a vibrant digital community through the voices of those most directly affected by issues of violence against Native women: Native women themselves. In this message, Deer offered to add some type of introductory 'warning' to emails containing particularly graphic information, and asked for members' opinions about this idea. She closed her message by thanking list members for their input and expressing her ongoing desire to see CAVNET_IW 'play a small part in the movement to end violence against Native women' (Message #4173).

The list members who responded to this message expressed gratitude for Deer's dedication to creating CAVNET_IW and for tirelessly posting information there that serves to witness and honour Indigenous women affected by violence, those who are survivors and those who are not. Responses also indicated list members' understanding that it is up to individual members to mediate their consumption and reception of traumatic stories or stories that have the potential to re-ignite trauma; it is not Deer's role, these members believe, to attempt to determine a hierarchy of disturbing information. 'Thanks for offering to place a 'warning,' on some of the emails,' writes Vicki Ybanez, an antiviolence advocate for Red Wing Consulting:

> I do think that it puts you in a difficult position of deciding what is too graphic or not. I would not want to ask you to do that and again refer to our personal responsibility in taking care of ourselves in this work. I find that some of the stories can be too hard for me in any given day. I make [a] decision about taking care of myself on that day and would not want to place that responsibility on anyone else. This is the nature of our work and I appreciate your offering news of what is happening to women in our communities! (Message #4177)

Lisa Brunner, Executive Director of the Community Resource Alliance Tribal Coalition, echoes Ybanez's sentiments about the value of CAVNET_IW in circulating narratives of trauma that would otherwise remain unheard by a larger public, and in utilizing these stories in her anti-violence activism. Like Ybanez, Brunner also recognises the long-term effects that can accrue for those, including Deer, who consistently read graphic descriptions of violence, and she also encourages individual members to take responsibility for their own emotional and psychic well-being. Brunner personalises her relationship with all Native women who have and do suffer from domestic and sexual violence by naming them as sisters, a move that configures CAVNET_IW as more than a community of internet 'users,' but as a family:

> I too appreciate Sarah's time and energy for keeping us informed of our stolen sisters, THEIR stories and how that impacts not just her family or community, but how [that] affects all of us. For Sarah to do this for us certainly cannot be an easy task and I for one am grateful that someone has taken [. . .] the time to search for our sisters. I use this information all the time in the work I do to educate about the violence against our women, I print out much of the stories and have them put in binders as an added resource. I learn so much from all of you in your

> comments and the stories you yourselves post. Communication is so important in all that we do as it also keeps us united in thought and at times like the murder of [Marisol], in prayer. My heart hurts to know she died in such a horrible violent way and to pray for her and her family is the trigger of reading HER story [...] I do not think Sarah needs to spend additional time censoring such stories. This is a listserv that addresses violence against Native women. Of course it will be graphic and bring about emotions from outrage to tears, but it also gives all the more reason to do what we do and fight harder for our people. I am sorry that [Lauren] is having a hard time with the realities that our women are facing every single day and the comments that come with that, and that she may take care of herself and take caution when opening a story about a stolen sister [capitals in original]. (Message #4178)

CAVNET_IW group members' responses clearly recognise the cumulative effects of reading traumatic narratives and working with Indigenous women affected by violence. As a locus for distilling much of this material over time, CAVNET_IW causes many list members to comprehend in a more quantifiable way the enormity of the circumstances Native women, their communities, and their anti-violence allies must constantly battle to achieve short and long-term successes. Deer's posting of individual news items in CAVNET_IW's virtual format disallows for the diffusion of traumatic narratives amidst other dissimilar news items as published within the print or online news sources in which these pieces originally appear. Thus, to read a series of CAVNET_IW postings on a given day or days is, often, to read a quantity of traumatic life stories back to back. 'I do recognize that the information is frequently tragic, graphic and scary,' wrote Diana in one of the final posts of the 'Posting of graphic information about Native women' thread:

> There are days that I sometimes feel overwhelmed but I am deeply committed to this work. The good in posting stories, articles, resources, etc., here outweighs any risk to my vicarious trauma, in my view, because I do then have an appreciation of the widespread impact of violence against women in Indian Country and get a significant understanding for how truly common and depraved it is. Violence is bad and it is getting worse. It is helpful to me to know that the ongoing viciousness to which all women, and especially native women, are exposed has significant daily impact on their lives and the lives of their children. This is why I have been in this business for twenty years and why I insist on knowing how dangerous the world really is for many native women. I deeply appreciate [Sarah's] time and effort in finding and posting these stories because for me in my work ignorance is not bliss—I must know about the violence in the world so that I can provide the level of service that my clients need without minimizing, avoiding, denying, rationalizing, or intellectualizing their experience. My defense mechanisms must be of a nature so that I can deal with my own emotional issues while not projecting my issues onto my clients. My knowledge of the violence to which they are exposed helps me understand, act, protect, advocate, and represent. I must know. (Message #4179)

Ultimately, it is story that is at the heart of all representation, and contestation over storytelling—whose gets told, by whom; whose is heard, by whom, where, and how—that impacts the representations of trauma experienced and narrated by Native North American women. In part because it is formatted into fractured news bytes and 'digestible' narrative chunks, mainstream news consistently undervalues and partially represents the circumstances of the violence that remains embedded in the fabric of contemporary Indigenous women's lives in the twenty-first century. CAVNET_IW negotiates the representations of loss and survivance, of chronic violence and unflagging efforts by survivors and advocates to stem the tide of this violence through grassroots activism and virtual community support. 'Nearly all of the Native women I know personally who are subscribers to CAVNET_IW are advocates with a history of personal victimization of themselves or family members,' notes Deer. 'It is rare to find a Native advocate whose life has not been personally touched by violence. Therefore, I view most posts to the list ([that] are not news articles) to be the voices of survivors' ('My responses'). In this way, CAVNET_IW demonstrates its flexibility as another 'promising example of the unique communicative advantage of virtuality: to be recruited as a relatively 'safe' refuge in which to begin the tentative process of community healing' (Landzelius 26), despite, or perhaps because of, occasional member debate around the ethical issues of the material that it posts. 'One of the challenges of communicating in this medium [of virtuality] is that sometimes we miss something in terms of tone/attitude when we can't talk directly—as is part of our culture as Native people,' Deer acknowledged to list members in her final message in the 'Posting of graphic information about Native women' thread. 'We will not all agree on tactics or even philosophy. But if we don't know where others stand it is impossible to facilitate collaboration' (Message #4216).

The project of circulating Native women's narratives of trauma through CAVNET_IW must delicately balance the multiple tasks of bearing witness to the past, fighting for activism in the present, and offering hope for future generations of Indigenous women and communities. The group strives to respect a diversity of Native people's values and worldviews, which in some communities has included traditional taboos around the direct discussion of sexual issues in specific contexts, including sexual violence. Yet CAVNET_IW gently insists upon recognising the historical changes that Indigenous communities have experienced that have led to the epic proportions of violence against Native women; part of this change is the gradual acceptance that the details of traumatic stories must sometimes be revealed and reiterated to be learned from and lessened, in the spirit of continuing tribal oral traditions.

As evidenced in the discussion thread above, most CAVNET_IW members understand the necessity of these changes as part of colonisation's ongoing legacy and of anti-violence activist resistance. 'It is critical that stories of our women and children are posted on CAVNET,' explains Brunner, 'otherwise they would continue to be invisible and their deaths going unnoticed by so many' ('RE: your remarks on CAVNET_IW'). In anti-violence workers' efforts to promote communal healing, Brunner believes that painful stories must emerge and be considered to affirm the empowered, respected roles of women in traditional Indigenous communities. 'That is why the listserv [CAVNET-IW] is important[,] so that we feel that impact and remember the sacred place in which our women are to be held and to be remembered regardless [of] how painful it may for us to read' ('RE: your remarks on CAVNET_IW). To diligently witness the trauma inflicted upon Indigenous women through CAVNET_IW may be, then, one significant step in moving closer to offering strategies for healing that trauma. 'One Alaska Native woman once told me (in person) that she views all Native women as survivors, even if they haven't personally been touched by violence,' Deer recalls. 'By nature of surviving mass murder and colonialisms, we are all survivors' ('My responses').

Notes

[1] Four significant pieces of legislation affecting the prosecution of sexual crimes on tribal lands are, in chronological order, The Major Crimes Act (1885), Public Law 280 (1953), The Indian Civil Rights Act (1968), and the Supreme Court Case of *Oliphant v. Suquamish Indian Tribe* (1978). For a concise summary of this legislation, see Sarah Deer 'Federal Indian Law and Violent Crime: Native Women and Children at the Mercy of the State' (20–22) and also, *Maze of Injustice* (28–30).

[2] Marc Dubin, Esq., former Special Counsel to the Office on Violence Against Women at the Justice Department, co-moderates CAVNET_IW with Deer, although Dubin acknowledges that he has 'no illusions about' the fact that it is Deer 'who is responsible for its success' (Marc Dubin, email to Jane Haladay. 29 December 2006).

[3] Citations of postings quoted from CAVNET_IW members will appear by message number as the messages are archived on the CAVNET_IW group site.

[4] Dubin founded CAVNET in 1996. For subscription and other information about this 'International Network of Anti-Violence Experts and Advocates,' see CAVNET's website at http://www.cavnet2.org/.

[5] 'Diana,' Message #4165, 11 April 2007. Identity withheld at author's request. All posts I quote in this thread are used with the permission of the authors, all of whom are identified with the exception of 'Diana,' who preferred to remain anonymous, and 'Lauren,' who unsubscribed from the list and thus could not be contacted for this article.

References

Brunner, Lisa. Message #4178. 13 April 2007.

——. 'RE: your remarks on CAVNET_IW.' Email to the author. 23 June 2007.

CAVNET_IW- CAVNET Indigenous Women (IW). 4 January 2007 <http://groups.yahoo.com/group/CAVNET_IW/>.

Deer, Sarah. 'Federal Indian Law and Violent Crime: Native Women and Children at the Mercy of the State.' *Social Justice: A Journal of Crime, Conflict, & World Order*. 31.4, Issue 98 (2004): 17–30.

——. Message #4173. 12 April 2007.

——. Message #4216. 20 April 2007.

——. 'My responses.' E-mail to the author. 7 January 2007.

'Diana.' Message #4170. 12 April 2007. Identity withheld at author's request.

——. Message #4179. 13 April 2007. Identity withheld at author's request.

Duran, Bonnie, Eduardo Duran, and Maria Yellow Horse Brave Heart. 'Native Americans and the Trauma of History.' *Studying Native America: Problems and Prospects*, ed. Russell Thornton. Madison: The University of Wisconsin Press, 1998. 64–76.

Gray, Nicole. Message #4184. 13 April 2007.

Landzelius, Kyra. *Native on the Net: Indigenous and Diasporic Peoples in the Virtual Age*. New York: Routledge, 2006.

'Lauren.' Message #4167. 11 April 2007. Author identity withheld.

Maze of Injustice: The failure to protect indigenous women from sexual violence in the USA. New York: Amnesty International USA (2007): 4. 10. Mar. 2007. <www.amnestyusa.org>.

Pasquet, Marissa. 'Woman Found Dead On Reservation Identified.' Message #4146. 5 April 2007.

'Poem.' Message #126. 16 January 2002.

Sanchez, Tawna. Message #4172. 12 April 2007.

Schaffer, Kay and Sidonie Smith. *Narrated Lives, Human Rights: The Ethics of Recognition*. New York: Palgrave Macmillan, 2004.

Smith, Andrea. *Conquest: Sexual Violence and American Indian Genocide*. Cambridge, MA: South End Press, 2005.

Ybanez, Vicki. Message #4171. 12 April 2007.

——. Message #4177. 12 April 2007.

Putting Site Back into Trauma Studies: A Study of Five Detention and Torture Centres in Santiago, Chile

Peter Read and Marivic Wyndham

At the end of the twentieth century it was possible to visit Berlin to observe the bombed church at Marienkirke in Kurfurstendamm and the bullet holes in the zoo buildings. You could visit the children's playground above Hitler's chancellery, the site of the 1933 book burning, the buildings which once held the Gestapo Headquarters, the Military High Command, the Air Ministry and Wansee where the Final Solution was discussed in 1942. All are visited regularly, most are included on official tours. In 1997 Martin Gilbert, a noted Holocaust historian, took a group of London postgraduate students on a 'holocaust journey'. Beginning in Berlin, they arrived at Number 4 Tiergartenstrasse, where the deaths of over 10,000 children were planned under the Nazi euthanasia program. Gilbert wrote,

> The enormity of the crime makes us pause, almost stop in our tracks. It is hard to comment on what was decided on here; hard, as we stand on the actual site, to react personally other than by silence and stillness. It takes a while before we are able to gather ourselves together—mentally as well as physically—and continue on our way. (25)

Curiously, not many of those Holocaust scholars trained in psychology or psychiatry significantly relate the site of violence to the psychotherapy of trauma victims. To heritage historians it seems a singular inattention. By excluding 'place' in what Dominick LaCapra calls the 'hauntingly possessive ghosts' of Holocaust survivors, and the 'empathetic unsettlement' of later generations, scholars set aside much recent research on the conjunction of trauma and site (xi; 102).[1] If British students, personally unconnected and two generations removed, could be thus overcome by visiting sites of actual or implied violence, what must be the effect of re-encountering sites of trauma among survivors, partners, children of survivors, the intimately connected from both sides?

Following the overthrow of Chile's Allende's government in 1973, Jorge Montealegre survived several months of torture and imprisonment at Chile's National Stadium. He returned to the site for the first time in 2001 to take part in a documentary.[2] Afterwards, he wrote:

> We would return to the stadium through memory. And it is not easy to unmake [that memory]. It remains here inside. The Stadium is a word which will always hold an echo in the galleries of memory. ... Nothing comparable to that state of Stadium which I have so often traversed through memory, where no one ages, where pain does not rule and cannot be pardoned. In memory I met myself, crouched under a blanket with the adolescent that I was. His orphanhood was confused with the orphanhood of the defeated, sharing the vulnerability of those left over. He had not realised that he was a survivor, until now, when he misses those of whom he writes: those who have died, the old ones who have lost their memory, those who have remained for ever in exile. (Montealegre 176)[3]

This paper is concerned with the correspondence between the profound trauma experienced by Chileans, and sites of imprisonment, interrogation, torture, disappearance and execution since Pinochet's seizure of power in 1973.[4]

A second limitation of Holocaust studies in relation to contemporary political trauma is the fraught environment in which the victims often subsequently must live. For West German Jews, in 1945, the war was over. Good had prevailed, evil was utterly vanquished. Retribution was accomplished, at least, to the satisfaction of some. Reconciliation with the perpetrators was scarcely an issue. Some survivors were able to begin to recover in remote and secure locations like the United States and Australia. Not so in the second half of the century where many supposedly post-trauma states remain unstable. Reconciliation cannot begin as long as the perpetrators believe that they have done no wrong, and the victims' and families of victims' pressing demands for 'truth and justice' remain generally unaddressed. Retribution remains impossible. In such parts of Asia, Africa and Latin America, tension may replace the terrorism of government or opponent, but trauma remains unresolved. Arjun Appadurai writes:

> The actions of various terrorist networks and agents seek to infuse all of everyday civilian life with fear. They presume a war where civilians do not exist. This is not just total war, as it has been waged by powerful states at different points of

> history, it is quotidian war, war as an everyday possibility, waged precisely to destabilise the idea that there is an 'everyday' for anyone outside the space and time of war. To this, terrorism adds the element of unpredictability, the key to producing constant fear. States that engage in this sort of strategy with respect to their own populations or other populations are rightly viewed as engaged in terrorism itself. (31–32)

In Chile, Following an unfavourable referendum, Pinochet stepped down as Commander-in-Chief of the Army in 1989; yet apprehension remained. In 1990 the incoming, moderate Aylwin government did not dare allow its National Commission on Truth and Reconciliation to name any of the perpetrators who had so terrorised the Chilean Left for seventeen years. Nor, indeed, did the armed forces concede that anything or anybody needed investigation. The National Security Council proposed to Aylwin:

> The army certainly sees no reason to seek pardon for having taken part in a patriotic labour. ... The Army of Chile solemnly declares that it will not accept being placed in the dock of the accused for having saved the freedom and sovereignty of the fatherland. (qtd. in Ensalaco 217)[5]

Terror and trauma continued to corrode Chilean public life. It was—and is—considered in bad taste to discuss the Pinochet terror; economic reconciliation was preferred to social, and personal testimonies seemed presented only by those who wanted to spoil the party (Valdés 4). The names and locations of most ex-centres of detention and torture vanished from much of Chilean society. Yet simultaneously a survivor of torture in the infamous Detention Centre 'Tejas Verdes' was imploring his compatriots to defend the past that they knew:

> If we, conscious of the terror which has been established in the country, pass through here without suspecting the existence of this place, what remains for those who want, deliberately, to deny the terror over the others. (Valdés 56)

The possibility of denial—much easier if the site of trauma has ceased to exist—alerts us to the third limitation of Holocaust therapists, preoccupied as they have understandably been, with the mental stability of survivors and their families. Family trauma, particularly for families of the disappeared, will continue for generations. National reconciliation should signify national stability—achieved in part through the alleviation of trauma. The future stability of states like Chile may turn on how trauma and terror are collectively, as well as individually, remembered and addressed.

Thus we return to the places of violence and execution. Sites may be destroyed, levelled and forgotten. They may be preserved, conserved and memorialised. They may carry no interpretation, minimal interpretation or one detailed and multifaceted. A trauma site may be made brutal, or serene, or, as we shall see, both of these things. But at every site lies conflict, and the possibility of further violence.

The five sites discussed here answer all these possibilities. Each contributes, or fails to contribute, to the alleviation of the collective and individual traumas which followed the seventeen years of terrorism by the Chilean state. The chapter argues for the inclusion of *site* in any exploration of trauma and its alleviation, for responsibility towards those involved beyond the survivors themselves, and for the centrality of the political milieu which follows the apparent overthrow of evil. Sites of great wickedness may become poetic and metaphysical terrains, but they also remain concrete and material where 'visible and invisible, past and present, physical and metaphysical come to exist and share a common space' (Tumarkin 233). For example, Montealegre carries the stadium in his memory forever (175).

Carrying it in Memory: The National Stadium

Between September and November 1973 more than fourteen thousand Chilean men and women were arrested and taken to the Stadium for interrogation, torture or execution. At this same symbolic site President Aylwin, succeeding Pinochet after the plebiscite which deposed him, made his inaugural address in 1990. Above the podium on the giant score-board, scrolled past the names of thousands of detained-disappeared.

The Stadium was the first large-scale detention centre used by the Pinochet terror. Most victims were summarily and violently arrested in the streets, factories, in universities, or in their homes. The purpose was to interrogate them as to their knowledge or membership of radical parties, especially the Movement of the Revolutionary Left (MIR), considered most likely to stage an immediate armed counter-coup. Many of the victims were blindfolded or blanketed, the majority were tortured, hundreds were killed and their bodies disposed of secretly. It may be that some of the bodies are buried within the grounds.

The fabric of the buildings remains almost untouched. A guide, clearly emotionally connected to the terrible events of September-November 1973 will conduct a tour for those who seek him out. He begins at the *Escotillas*, the entrances into the main stadium in which men were herded, and often killed. Small calibre bullets are still lodged in the walls, but the prisoners' inscriptions are indecipherable beneath the white-wash applied by soldiers before the Army withdrew. Apart from some 1990s football-fan graffiti, these amenities have not been touched since the coup. The areas in the tour, it seems, have been listed for preservation in the national estate, but neither conservation nor curating has begun. The tour continues of bathrooms into which dozens of men were crammed, the washbasins encrusted in calcium decades old. Here, to these clothes racks in the changing rooms, prisoners were tied. It was at this very spot that the *encapuchado*, the hooded identifier of the members of the revolutionary left, pointed out those then immediately scheduled for torture and death. From the highest roof above the press gallery, just up there, certain prisoners, handcuffed and blindfolded, were ordered to 'fly' by drunken soldiers seeking amusement. The tour leaves the main stadium building. Women prisoners were held in the changing rooms of the swimming pool complex. Steps lead downwards to the filthy dark, cold and damp. The florescent lights are rusting, the toilets are black. Many women prisoners, returning to the stadium, cannot bear to re-enter their place of humiliation and torture. Here, outside the stadium, the Red Cross, foreign press and human rights investigators were temporarily camped; but this road to the left led only to death, and the prisoners knew it. The guide follows it in somber silence, half a kilometre to the infamous Velodrome, whose entrance passage is pocked with dozens of bullets. Each one, probably, represents a merciful death. Though the prisoners' last words have been crudely erased, a message, inscribed only two weeks after the death of the dictator in 2006 reads,

> Pinochet, responsible for the death of many persons
> Let us not forget it.

The tour ends in the weightlifting room, where the screams of the tortured, which so terrorise the memory of the survivors, could not be easily heard. It is here that the central monument to the detained-disappeared will be placed.

What information, what signage will accompany the site-exhibition, in a country where open discussion of the Pinochet years is still almost universally, and voluntarily, proscribed? What will be omitted in the interpretation of the bullet-marked stadium in this trauma-ridden and unstable country? We cannot be sure that conservation will take place at all. A major bi-centenary project to upgrade the Stadium and its grounds, scheduled for completion by 2010, may overtake other priorities. The historically curious may call upon the 'Museum of Communist Treachery' in Djakarta, but within the Indonesian archipelago there is not one memorial to the more than 500,000 left-wing Indonesians killed in the 1950s.[6] In former East Germany, World War II monuments stressed the suffering of the communists and belittled the Shoah, while in West Germany, memorialising tended to name neither the victims nor the perpetrators until the 1980s. Only in recent decades have memorials been erected at specific sites of execution, and the victims named. Individual Nazis, however, are still seldom identified (Neumann 113; 258–61). The Spanish Government since 2006 allows compensation for victims of the Civil War, but not prosecution of the perpetrators (Boletín Oficial).

Clearly the National Stadium of Chile will be interpreted differently by left and right, young and old survivors and those who did not experience its horrors. Among the survivors, anguish and trauma remains unresolved. Montealegre reflects,

> In another documentary I see myself visiting the stadium with my sister. In front of an *escotilla* I try to express what I have clumsily tried to say or avoid saying. It's curious. Before the cameras we survivors relate what the others can no longer relate. We talk for ourselves, but knowing that we are explaining a collective

> moment. We speak for the others. We are everybody and nobody. And we tell it urgently because the survivors of any time are naturally a species-in-extinction. But the documentaries will survive us marvelously. In these we are the people of yesterday, and the people of before-yesterday. Fragments of mirrors making markers for the future. (172)

People of Yesterday: Villa Grimaldi

Villa Grimaldi was one of the first, and among the most infamous, of the torture/detention centres constructed to hold the multitude of new arrests in the capital. It is here that the tension between the purposes of creating a serene haven for the survivors, and the education of those who need to be informed and in a sense traumatised, are most raw: fresh lawns and rusty barbed wire are juxtaposed in a manner not universally admired even by the constructors of the memorial.[7]

Villa Grimaldi was a graceful nineteenth-century estate of some five hectares on the then outskirts of Santiago. The military seized the main building and modified the interior of the water tower at the rear of the estate as a prison and execution chamber. Both were demolished by the secret intelligence service, the DINA, when it left, but the tower has been reconstructed. The principal restoration and reconstruction has been carried out by successive Chilean Governments and completed in May 2007.

The first impression to the visitor is of serenity and peace. The entrance sign reads:

> Villa Grimaldi Peace Park
> Secret Centre of Detention, Torture and Extermination between 1973 and 1979
> 4 500 tortured
> 226 detained disappeared and executed
>
> To our visitors:
> This place is a memorial
> Visit it with respect
> It holds a long history which belongs to us all
> Let us care for it that it may endure and teach us

Villa Grimaldi is also a place of memorialisation for many leftist political groups. The signage erected by the Centre for Truth and Justice is emotionally much sharper:

> Life passed through here, with its songs, flags and ideals.
>
> Here remain the dreams of Liberty and Justice of Juan, Luis, Manuel and of such other compañeros

> The memories give us strength to follow in search of truth and justice
> Forever forward brothers in dreams and utopias

Note how the government signage requires mourning rather than 'truth and justice'. Indeed, the very design of the park reflects the difficult course taken here, and nationally, between the cautious state seeking retribution only in the courts, the traumatised individual survivors who mostly seek peace, and the grieving families who also want the young to understand what happened. Juxtaposed are the sweet soft lawns, a model of the former villa, the flower beds, a rose in memory of each woman who died here, the limpid fountain, the graceful interior stone walls, the outdoor theatre, the contemplative benches, above all, the garden's imbued serenity. The anguish and trauma is reflected in the brutal cement wall standing at the rear of the park, the DINA's ugly preserved entrance gate, the angry signage demanding justice, the reconstruction of the one metre-square 'cells' and torture chambers in the tower in which prisoners were held, and a collection of recovered railway sleepers to which prisoners were tied and thrown into the sea from helicopters. The third element is the wrenching emotions of lives so horribly lost. The Sala de la Memoria (the Memory Room) holds photographs and tiny mementoes of some of the disappeared. Michelle Peña, eight months pregnant, gave her niece three little mementoes as she departed for a rally at the University of Technology (USACH) from which she never returned. A survivor, now acting as guide, recalls how officers' wives and children, splashing in the villa's pool, could clearly hear the screams from the tower, but somehow subsumed the screams of the tortured and the screams of the swimming children into the same aural ambience.

Indonesian Hindus had powerful rituals to cleanse the places of traumatic public death from which souls who died in the Bali bombing might be released. Not so Chileans who must rely mostly on civil procedures to cleanse the site and release souls. Yet the state is unwilling. Only a handful of perpetrators of state terror are today imprisoned, and while the guilty remain unpunished, trauma remains unrequited. The Chilean state appears to prefer what Colin Tatz has called organised forgetting. The traumatised, abandoned by the state,

> must forgo the desire or need for retributive justice; it is they who must eschew notions of guilt and atonement, and, all too often, forgo compensation for harms done. It is they who must agree to the diminution, or even abolition, of that shared historical memory which holds victims groups together. It is they who must concur in the substitution of their memory and their history by our history. It is they who must connive at ignoring the importance of accountability for the crimes committed against them, and agree to the blurring and obliteration of responsibility for who did what to them. It is they who must cease being so hysterical about denialism, the major tributary of forgetting which claims that there was anything to remember in the first place. (Tatz 11–13)

Apologists for the mildly worded Villa Grimaldi entrance sign might defend their position, by asking, like Australia's Archbishop Penman arguing against the possible prosecution of Nazi war criminals living in Australia, 'are we a nation of mercy and forgiveness or one of vengeance?' (Tatz 29).

Forgiveness or Vengeance: Jose Domingo Cañas

Jose Domingo Cañas is a street containing another centre rivalling Villa Grimaldi in infamy. The prison takes its name from this address. It was one of several centres run by the Directorate of National Intelligence, the DINA. All the buildings on the site were destroyed by a toy manufacturer which had bought the site as an extension of its own premises next door, for no better motive, it is alleged, than to discourage it becoming a national monument. But a monument it became.

In recent years Jose Domingo Cañas has been an empty wasteland of half an acre used as a carpark. At first sight, not much distinguishes it from any demolition site awaiting development save a monument on the street, and the murals and graffiti inscribed on the two longer walls separating the site from the toy factory and a private house on the other side. But what murals!

The view of the Advisory Board of National Monuments is represented on the street monument. 'Jose Domingo Cañas' is described as a 'House of Torture':

In this house No. 1367 Jose Domingo Cañas
In the year 1974 during the
Military dictatorship (1973–1990) were
42 detained-disappeared compañeros

The victims are then identified. But a poetic rather than militant inscription on each side of the obelisk points to the government's difficulty in balancing the nation's political forces.

No such ambiguity troubles the political organisations whose members were tortured here and killed in the 1970s. These groups, representing shanty towns or workers' collectives, were accorded the right to inscribe their own messages. Strongest of all in language and feeling is that of the Pedro Rojas Brigade from the radical shanty town of La Legua:

Here were committed
The most ferocious violations
Of human dignity

And for this reason we demand
Justice and Punishment
For the torturers

A painting of hands beneath a waterfall pointing towards the rising sun carries the caption:

The fallen . . .
Eternal fountains
Of life

A graphic painting of a naked man and woman tied by the hands to a cell roof:

Here
was murdered
The flesh
But not
The idea

On another section of the original prison perimeter fence:

We do not forget
We do not forgive

A wrenching depiction of the metre-square prisoner cages reads:

This was a nightmare

From the shanty town of La Victoria:

we were
we are we will be

A verse of M. Carvalho:

Even after death
I will keep on giving my testimony
of death. This motionless rain [the mural]
will be me spitting

Masked, though, beneath the fury and despair of the murals lie the deeper traumas of the families of the tortured. Victims have asked their therapists or friends,

> How can I make love to my wife, when I have seen her be raped? Why can't she defend herself more? Can she love me and understand that I couldn't help her?

Or:

> When my husband asked me to give information did he do it to protect us or because he betrayed his ideals? Can I respect him after this?

Or:

> Can my son respect me after he has seen me like that? (Agger and Jensen 121)[8]

An inability to make closure follows every state disappearance. Partners lived first through a deadly uncertainty. Hebe de Bonafine, mother of an Argentinian disappeared described a crippling anxiety for her son whom she could not help:

> Many of us found out where they were held, how they were tortured, what instruments they used, the names of the torturers, where they lived. Slowly we reconstructed the events. Every day we heard new stories and the news got worse. We began to hear words like *capucha, submarine, picana* and we began to piece together the full extent of the horror. All this changes you. It changes your values. It changes the way you think. (Fisher 66)

Sol Sierra, President in 2002 of the Association of the Families of the Detained-Disappeared, reported 200 members of her association who had died from unknown illnesses and the grief and sense of impotence they had been living with. No period of bereavement, mourning and healing could follow a disappearance without trace. The missing person was both alive and dead. The intense suffering could find no relief. When a newly discovered body was about to be identified, the family would hope it was not their loved one—also hope that it was. Eventually a woman might decide that her husband must be dead and that life must somehow go on; it was as if that she had herself killed him, not the state. Disappearances were rarely spoken of at home while a lingering anxiety and insecurity generated a progressively greater isolation in suffering. Children endured different sufferings, or might take on the burden of making up for a parent's unfulfilled life. Often they grew isolated as maturing adults. Sierra wrote:

> [. . .] they come to the stage of their life between twenty five and thirty years old [. . .] A depression comes on them, a psychological disorder. We have nearly twenty cases irrecoverable of schizophrenia in children of the disappeared. The doctors cannot explain it . . . all of a sudden they suffer some crisis as a result of this abnormal situation they have been living, a crisis that causes them a psychological disturbance so great that they have become schizophrenic. (qtd. in Salimovich and Weinstein 72–89)

Grief and rage often followed the belated news of an execution or a body identified, then active denial and feelings of impotence. Fear became the organising principle of life.[9]

Paralysing trauma among the families continued long after the destruction of the armed revolutionary left and the disbanding of the hated DINA in the middle 1976. To protest at places like Jose Domingo Cañas at any point during the dictatorship was an act of considerable courage. The Danish psychotherapists Inger Agger and Soren Jensen arrived at another Santiago torture centre in 1989 just as an illegal protest was about to begin. They were told to give their exact names and passport numbers to their friends; to look for a place to protect them from water cannon; to hold a slice of lemon to their noses against tear gas; to run towards the police, not away from them; when the protest was over they were to disband pretending to be tourists. Minutes later, and before the police had arrived in any numbers, the demonstration was over:

> The passers-by pick up, read and put the pamphlets in their pockets and bags, and seconds later the traffic is moving again. The demonstrators have disappeared. If the banners had not still been on the wall and the pamphlets in our pockets, we would not have been sure that this had really happened. (Agger and Jensen 1–2)

When the Banner Disappears off the Wall: Londres 38

On 3 January 2007 a group of thirty protesters held their weekly vigil outside the former torture and disappearance centre, 38 London Street. They arranged the candles along the footpath; they pasted pictures of a dozen of the 384 people who had been disappeared from Londres 38.[10] They sang, they made speeches, they chatted to each other, they erected the banner:

Londres 38
(ex House of Torture and Murder)
House of Memory
Collective 119[11]

As evening fell they removed the banner but left the photographs stuck on the wall of the building. Some time during the night, workers employed by the building's management covered the photographs with whitewash. Next morning nothing remained of the protest. The photographs of the disappeared had themselves disappeared.

Londres 38 is occupied by the Instituto O'Higgiano, intimately connected with the Chilean Army. The government has not thought it wise to use force to evict them, nor managed to persuade them to exchange this prime mid-city site for another. Officials do not welcome enquiries. In the 1990s they repainted the building's street number as Number 40 in a futile attempt to misdirect visitors. But everyone involved in the protest movement knows where it is. Someone, perhaps from Collectivo 119, has tried to remove the new number altogether.

Londres 38 is a site where denial is strong and the possibility of healing is weak. What remains of the cells, the instruments of torture? Are the walls upstairs, like those of the stadium *escotillas*, bullet-holed, are the last inscriptions of prisoners still engraved on the walls of the cells? What remains of the torture instruments—the containers of water, urine and excrement into which prisoners' heads were forced, the desperately tiny cages, the *picana* (electric cattle prod), the *parilla*, the 'grill', a metal frame which connected to a generator and handle to vary the voltage. It seems unlikely that the O'Higgins society will leave any traces. Torture victims face an eternal denial of their sufferings.

Hernán Valdés was tortured at the Tejas Verdes centre. He describes his first torture session:

> One of them approaches me, takes two points of the hood and makes a very strong knot under the bridge of my nose so that the middle of the face remains uncovered for them. One coils a cable around the big toes of my damp feet. There is a very brief silence and next I feel a tickling sensation up to my knees. I scream, more than anything, out of fear. They insult me, as if scandalized by my delicacy. I feel a movement of air at my side and someone gives me with all the force he's capable of, a punch in the pit of the stomach. It's like they have cut me in two. For a fraction of a second I lose consciousness. I recover because I'm on the point of asphyxiation. Someone rubs me violently on the heart. . . . I start to breathe through the mouth at a diabolical rate. I can't get any air. My breast heaves, my ribs like a grating squeezing me. Nothing remains of me but this hysterical greed in my breast to swallow air.
>
> What's your name? . . .
> Her—nán Val—déz I manage to let out in various spaces. I receive a blow with a rubber club, from behind, on the shoulder.
> 'Sir', *huevón*, [motherfucker] more respect!
> They begin to ask all the facts of my membership, quickly, facts which they should have there, on a card. . . . I give answers, rapidly, without recovering breath, 'Single, sir', 'One metre sixty five, sir' etcetera.
> Colour of eyes?
> Chestnut, sir.
> A jolt of the current goes up my bones up to the knees.
> What do you mean, 'chestnut'? *huevón*, Coffee it will be.
> Coffee, sir.
> Colour of hair?
> Coffee, sir.
> Another jolt of the current. The guys laugh. It is not exactly pain which the electricity produces, but a brutal internal shaking which strips the bones naked.
> So you're a fag.
> No sir
> Why not? Here it's written that you're a fag.
> It is another voice. I don't manage to ask where it is written. This time a jolt of the current practically knocks my feet from under me and I fall to the cement floor. Instantly they make me rise, kicking me. I don't know how I manage it. [. . .]

Valdés' description continues for another ten pages. Later in the same session, under increasingly excruciating sexual electrical torture, he is forced to describe his writings, the whereabouts of certain people, even his girlfriend's genital organs (117–19).

The passage reveals many of the most hateful features of the regime of Chilean torture: an equal emphasis on the humiliation of the mental, the sexual, the physical and the psychic, implemented and approved as an official instrument of intimidation by the regime.[12] Valdés' testimony gives a tiny indication of that from which Chilean torture victims have struggled to recover. The effects involve what Agger and Jensen describe as an existential crisis which may involve protecting the self at the cost of others, a psychic numbing from which it may be difficult to return, confusion between fantasy and reality, extreme fear after release, a perception of inferiority, guilt and betrayal, an inability to speak about the experience, shame, identification with the aggressor, loss of sexual desire, self-destruction or self harm, self loathing, destruction of intimate relationships, and gastric, respiratory and cardio-vascular psychosomatic symptoms. They summarise the symptoms afflicting torture victims as:

> how to bring the hidden self out of its shelter and handle the affective distress following the reduction of psychic numbing. When the hidden self no longer protects the survivor by staying in its shelter, she or he is also faced with the task of finding a bearable solution to the problem of complicity. In other words, how is the split-off memory fragment integrated, and how is a connection to life re-established? (Agger and Jensen 90–101)

How much more difficult will be the return to an integrated personality when an arm of the state, located at Londres 38, continues to deny that torture ever occurred there?

Re-establishing a Connection to Life: Loyola/Neptuno

A large armed-services camp which also, in the final years of the regime, served as a torture and detention centre was situated in the working-class suburb of Lautaro. Much less is known of its activities. It is included in this excoriating research because most of its original structures still exist, even the cells. Torture instruments and prisoners' graffiti may even also be preserved underground. Here the state, heritage professionals, families of the disappeared, the tortured and survivors, possibly even the descendants of the perpetrators, have a chance. In a marginally more receptive political climate, they may have an opportunity to develop a new and truthful historical display. But what is new? What is truth? And for which Chilean generations?

For most of the twentieth century the United States heritage industry suffered from slavery-amnesia. In the interpretations of most museums, Civil War soldiers fought to save the Union rather than to end slavery. Tour guides of southern mansions referred to 'servants', slave quarters were not part of the tour. Guilt and shame seemed to prevent a more open discussion. The attitudes of 'middle America' began to change only after television and film spectaculars like *Roots* and *Amistad*. Recently, possible reparations and an apology to African Americans have become topical issues—nearly a century and a half after the end of the Civil War. Yet what should replace the ideology of 'moonlight and magnolias' to reflect the long trauma of African suffering? The plantation as a death-centric institution? The universal violation of human rights? The triumph of the 'Underground Railway' escape route to Canada? A catalogue of evils? A bridge to reconciliation? Magnification of the way in which slaves refashioned themselves culturally and economically? The triumph of the African-American in the face of insuperable odds? How, asks the heritage historian Francis Ruffins, should one speak to new generations who are the descendants both of victims *and* victimisers (396–434)?

LaCapra refers to these new generations as in need of an 'empathetic unsettlement' which 'may take different forms, and may at times result in secondary or muted trauma' (102). Loyola/Neptuno then, offers the possibility to educate those who have been taught nothing, so that they may be traumatised, then de-traumatised in offering a form of reconciliation between the descendants of all the protagonists in this most hateful and desperate conflict.

Conflicting memories among the protagonists is the first obstacle. Reconciliation will not be easy in their lifetime. In Poland, memorials have been utilised to preserve what the dominant (non Jewish) group wants to remember; what it wants to forget is 'destroyed, neglected or preserved in a distorted way'. The name 'Ghetto Victims' only appears rather rarely in memorials in Polish towns. The communist regime insisted on the equation of communism with the long Polish struggle for independence. The historian Slawomir Kaprallski writes: 'The Jews were eliminated physically by the Nazis; the memory of the Jews has been eliminated systematically by the Poles' (46). The spectacle will be familiar to those who have seen the photographs of the disappeared themselves disappear each week from the walls of Londres 38. Reconcilation may not be possible for several generations. In 2000, descendants of victims and perpetrators walked side by side for the first time to a memorial to Aborigines massacred at Myall Creek in New South Wales: one hundred and sixty two years after the event (Read, 'The Truth That Will Set Us All Free'). In the Greek village of Drakeia 116 men were massacred by Nazis in late 1944 following the killing of two German soldiers by Partisans. For decades, depending in part on the left-right oscillation of Greek politics, blame has been apportioned to partisans, communists, quiescent villagers and to a variety of individuals—but hardly ever to the Nazis themselves. The terrible legacy of blame and counter-blame to some is worse than the massacre itself (Van Boeshoten). Yet an insistence on forced remembering may also be counter-productive. A German woman daily walking in streets named after the village children killed by the Nazis responded:

> On the one hand I think it's a good idea to remember it. On the other hand, I don't think it's all that good for me that I am constantly reminded of it, because I didn't have anything to do with it. ... Because that always affects me, and because I then think about how terrible that was, and again and again am reminded of how terrible it was. And of what the children must have experienced. ... Our generation has actually got nothing to do with it, but we are now being burdened with it here. (Neumann 214)

The question of what *might* be presented at Loyola/Neptuno slides to—what historical interpretation: is it *possible* empathetically to unsettle younger Chileans? The Drakeia researcher Riki Van Boeschoten concludes that interpretation depends to a large extent on the pre-existing culture of the society in question (46–48). Just so. We should remind ourselves of the critical nature of the political in any attempt either to educate or to de-traumatise the present or future generations. Agger and Jensen—the trauma therapists studying the Chilean experience—conclude:

> To therapists working in democratic countries with a history of many years of peace, the importance of the relationship between politics and psychology is difficult to grasp. Under state terrorism this position is taken for granted. [...] Only afterwards did we appreciate the impact of this dimension for the understanding of trauma. Therefore, we must again emphasize the words of the Chilean psychologist who said that 'if you cannot work with this aspect, people will never really improve'. (208)

Whatever is decided, the raw materials of Loyola/Neptuno bear an infinite capacity to stun young people, like those at Number 4 Tiergarten, into silence and stillness. They are all here: the soldiers' parade ground, the machinery shed, the barracks, the watch-towers, the flag pole, the barbed wire, the enclosing wall, the guard house, the officers' quarters, the main-gate key board still labelled with the keys for certain vehicles and entrances, the insignia of the last regiment to occupy the barracks, the safe. And the cells; they have apparently not been destroyed, but remain as a dozen flights of stairs disappearing below the cement parade ground filled with building rubble to prevent entrance. Perhaps the army destroyed the cells before they filled the entrances with rubble. It seems unlikely.

Recovery in Chile will be very slow. Sulphurous hatreds and traumas burn slowly beneath a thin façade of unity. Pinochet's desire, expressed in his 1978 General Amnesty, to 'leave behind hatreds' and to 'promote national reunification' seems impossible among the direct participants. The children of the military and of the victims find it hardest to foresee national reconciliation (Andreani and Cerda 221). It is the succeeding generation which will require the evidence of the preserved sites of torture, detention and disappearance to heal their nation's trauma.

We may agree with Cathy Caruth that trauma 'does not easily serve as a record of the past but precisely registers the force of an experience that is not yet fully owned' (151). Contemporary Chile does not offer reassurance that the national experience will soon be owned by anyone. Those sympathetic to an honest historical display at the stadium have been waiting for four years for conservation (funded by charity, not the government) to begin. The collective and families supporting memorialisation at Jose Domingo Cañas are fighting a losing battle with the department of Urban Housing over the future of the site. Londres 38 remains an enigma of hostile denial. Rumours circulate that Urban Housing has recently taken control of Loyola/Neptuno and may begin soon to 'develop' the site. Only Villa Grimaldi remains a genuine, state-sponsored memorial to a violent and vicious past, but the park, perhaps because it is the only memorial, bears too many conflicting interpretations of trauma and history.

Ariel Dorfman was a pro-Allende supporter forced into exile. His play *Death and the Maiden* depicts the post-Pinochet conflict between a pro-justice lawyer, his wife, a torture victim, and a doctor who was present at her torture. He presents the prospect of reconciliation thus:

> How can those who tortured and those who were tortured exist in the same land? How to heal a country that has been traumatized by repression if the fear to speak out is still omnipresent everywhere? And how do you reach the truth if lying has become a habit? How do we keep the past alive without becoming its prisoner? How do we forget it without becoming its prisoner? Is it legitimate to sacrifice the truth to insure peace? And what are the consequences of suppressing that past and the truth it is whispering or howling to us? Are people free to search for justice and equality if the threat of a military intervention haunt them? ... And perhaps the greatest dilemma of them all: how to confront these issues without destroying the national consensus, which creates democratic stability. (Dorfman 73)

These seem to us to be the central questions facing Chile today.

Notes

[1] Examples of writings on environmental loss include Peter Read, *Returning to Nothing*; Sylvia Hood Washington, Paul Rosier, and Heather Goodall, *Echoes from the Poisoned Well*.

[2] The documentary is *Estadio Nacional*, directed and produced by Carmen Luz Parot.

[3] The blankets in the title and in the passage refer to the blankets thrown over prisoners' heads to prevent them identifying their surroundings or accusers.

[4] The Chilean Commission of Investigation into state terrorism committed during Pinochet's years of office (1973–89). The 'Rettig Report' names some 30,000 victims of torture and 3,000 disappearances or executions ("Informe de la comisión Nacional").

[5] A. Pinochet Ugarte, 'Respuestas de las Fuerzas Armadas y de Orden', 27 March 1991 (Ensalaco 217).

[6] Seminar discussion at the University of Sydney with Prof. Adrian Vickers; see also Denis Byrne.

[7] The tension is conveyed in the title of a conference *A Museum in Villa Grimaldi for the Memory and Education in Human Rights*, Corporación Parque de la Paz Villa Grimaldi, Municipalidad de Peñalolén, 2005.

[8] Agger and Jensen citation of D. Becker, M. Castillo, R. Dominguez, 'Tortura y Daño en La Familia', 1987.

[9] Sierra in S. Salimovich and E. Weinsten (72–89; 82–83); see also Mark Ensalaco (232); and E. Perel and J. Saul (135–52).

[10] This passive form of the verb 'to disappear' entered the language via Latin America in the 1970s. 'Londres 38' signifies 38 London Street.

[11] An individual collective takes responsibility for the maintenance of appropriate action at a number of sites in Santiago. Collective 119 takes its name from the 119

people falsely named by the government as having escaped to, and been killed in Argentina.

[12] See also the 1974 Amnesty International Report *Torture as Official Policy in Chile*.

References

Agger, Inger, and Soren Jensen. *Trauma and Healing Under State Terrorism*. London: Zed, 1996.

Amnesty International. *Torture as Official Policy in Chile*. London: Amnesty International, 1974.

Andreani, María, and Mariane Cerda. 'El Si-No de la Reconciliación. Representaciones Sociales de la Reconciliación en los Jóvenes.' Fundación Documentación y Archivo de la Vicaría de la Solidaridad, 2000.

Appadurai, Arjun. *Fear of Small Numbers*. Durham: Duke, 2006.

Boletín Oficial de Las Cortes Generales, Ley 24/2006 [Spain].

Byrne, Denis. 'The Archaeology of Disaster.' *Public History Review* 5.6 (1996–97): 17–29.

Caruth, Cathy, ed. *Trauma, Explorations in Memory*. Baltimore: Johns Hopkins, 1995.

Chile. Ministerio del Interior. *Informe de la Comisión Nacional sobre Prisión Politica y Tortura*. Santiago: Gobierno de Chile, 1991.

Corporación Parque de la Paz Villa Grimaldi. *A Museum in Villa Grimaldi for the Memory and Education in Human Rights*. Corporación Parque de la Paz Villa Grimaldi: Municipalidad de Peñalolén, 2005.

Dorfman, Ariel. *Death and the Maiden*. New York: Penguin, 1991.

Ensalaco, Mark. *Chile Under Pinochet*. Philadelphia: U of Pennsylvania P, 2000.

Fisher, Jo. *Mothers of the Disappeared*. Boston: South End Press, 1989.

Gilbert, Martin. *Holocaust Journey*. London: Weidenfeld and Nicholson, 1997.

Kaprallski, Slawomir. 'Battlefields of Memory: Landscape and Memory in Polish-Jewish Relations.' *History and Memory* 13 (2001): 35–50.

LaCapra, Dominick. *Writing History, Writing Trauma*. Baltimore: Johns Hopkins, 2001.

Luz Parot, Carmen. *Estadio Nacional*. Dir. and Prod. Carmen Luz Parot. Chile, 2001.

Montealegre, Jorge. *Frazadas del Estadio Nacional* [Blankets of the National Stadium]. Colección Septiembre, 2003.

Neumann, klaus. Shifting Memories: the Nazi past in the New Germany. Ann Arbour: University of Michigan Press, 2000.

Perel, E., and J. Saul. 'A Family Therapy Approach to Holocaust Survivor Families.' *Healing Their Wounds. Psychotherapy with Holocaust Survivors and Their Families*. Ed. Paul Marcus and Alan Rosenberg. New York: Praeger, 1989. 135–52.

Read, Peter. *Returning to Nothing*. Melbourne: Cambridge UP, 1996.

——. 'The Truth That Will Set Us All Free: An Uncertain History of Memorials to Indigenous Australians.' *The Many Faces of Denial*. Ed. Graham Dawson and Louise Purbrick. Palgrave, 2007. NYP.

Ruffins, Francis D. 'Revisiting the Old Plantation: Reparations, Reconciliation, and Museumizing American Slavery.' *Museum Frictions*. Ed. Ivan Karp, Corinne Kratz, Lyn Szwaja, and Tomás Ybarra-Frausto. Durham: Duke, 2006. 394–434.

Salimovich, S., and E. Weinstein. 'Victims of Fear: The Social Psychology of Repression.' *Fear at the Edge: State Terror and Resistance in Latin Americas*. Ed. Juan Corradi, Patricia Weiss Fagen, and Manuel Antonio Garretón. Berkeley: U of California, 1992. 72–89.

Tatz, Colin. 'Reflections on the Politics of Remembering and Forgetting.' Centre for Comparative Genocide Studies. Sydney: Macquarie U, 1994.

Tumarkin, Maria. *Traumascapes*. Carlton: Melbourne UP, 2005.

Valdés, Hernán. *Tejas Verdes*. Santiago: LOM Ediciones, 1996.

Van Boeschoten, Riki. 'Broken Bonds and Divided Memories: Wartime Massacres Reconsidered in a Comparative Perspective.' *Oral History* 35.1 (2007): 39–48.

Washington, Sylvia Hood, Paul Rosier, and Heather Goodall. *Echoes from the Poisoned Well*. Lanham: Lexington Books, 2006.

Textual Traumata: Letters to Lindy Chamberlain

Deborah Staines

How societies remember, Paul Connerton tells us, is physically embodied through ritual and performance, habit and memory.[1] In addition, what societies choose to remember and how they interpret those memories, is crucial to what will be recognised as *traumatic* memory. Here, I will look at one instance where a traumatic event within the life of a family enters the circuits of social and cultural construction that enable pain and suffering to be collectively understood as 'cultural trauma'.[2] Although it may seem to be self evident which events will be defined as cultural trauma (such as natural disasters or genocide), the case study in this article will consider an event where the incorporation of individual trauma into a larger manifestation of collective trauma was by no means a given: the Chamberlain Case, in which the disappearance of an infant, the conviction of her mother for murder, and the divisive ramifications of these events affected an entire nation. How and why did this event assume these proportions? The life writing that emerged around the case is important to answering this question, as well as raising more general questions about the development of collective trauma.

Trauma has grown into a substantial medicalised category of human experience that exceeds strictly clinical parameters. Contextualising my arguments here, are a variety of disciplinary uses of trauma theory across the humanities and social sciences, and in legal practice a valuing of affective side-effects from violent crime.[3] Increasingly the vulnerability of society and culture—as well as individuals—to traumatic episodes is theorised as cultural trauma. This is a term that focuses on the collective aspects of trauma resulting from atrocity, disaster and grief, and the struggle to integrate an event personally and collectively. This re-classification of certain historical events and resulting conditions as traumatic not only to individuals but more broadly to society and culture involves processes of transmission variously described as: inherited trauma, transgenerational trauma, national trauma, social trauma, collective trauma, and cultural trauma.[4] Although each of these terms has its own subtle distinctions, they are all representative of attempts to describe a kind of embedded and permanent damage to a society and its culture. This marks trauma as more than a clinical episode within the confines of an individual life. It evokes a society struggling to integrate an event and continuing to relive it—a notion that remains contentious even though it is by now broadly applied. In a range of discourses, the tropes of trauma are used to imagine and interpret aspects of cultural change. We readily see this in the various forms and manifestations of trauma theory: used to deconstruct a literary work, to explain the cultural productions of second and third generations as post-traumatic, or when it is extended to describe the experience of collectivities as cultural trauma.

The main exponents of the term cultural trauma are the sociologists associated with the Yale School, and in particular Jeffrey Alexander, through his publications on cultural trauma, social performance, and collective identity. The kinds of events which have been distinguished as cultural trauma include the Holocaust, African-American slavery, war, and the Argentine disappeared. As Alexander explains it, the collective adoption of an event as a cultural trauma is not random—it is the result of strategic efforts to represent particular events as crucial to society at large, and evidenced with historical material. His deployment of the term addresses collective aspects of individual trauma resulting from atrocity, disaster and grief, described as an element of collective identity. To be classified as a cultural trauma, the effects must be seen to extend beyond an individual, and indeed, the injury must be recognised as having been sustained by a collective. Alexander's systematic analysis, 'Toward a Theory of Cultural Trauma', identifies a structured negotiation and mediation of cultural trauma, presented in this model:

- claims made by agents/carrier groups, e.g. victims, activists, elites, media
- reception of claims by the broader community

- working through claims in cultural domains, e.g. church, family, state, courts, professions
- re-classification of events as a cultural trauma, and circulation of a new historical narrative attesting to this.[5]

This model proposes that at the cultural level, the mechanisms of trauma transmission involve social agents and contending groups making representations and claims. From this perspective, Neil Smelser suggests cultural traumas are seen to be 'made, not born' and the definition and transmission of cultural trauma by 'cultural carriers' such as intellectuals, politicians, journalists, and community leaders is vital (38). Through mediation in the public sphere—through listening to testimonies, seeing documentary photographs, watching dramatisations—a new historical narrative emerges from debate, and so an event is (re)defined, recognised, and adopted as part of the collective history (i.e. of a city, nation, region). In Alexander's model of the processing of cultural trauma, the work of cultural carriers draws on and rearticulates prevalent trauma tropes. The work of the cultural carriers, imbued by a politics of recognition, shapes the new narrative, and explains in part why some events are recognised as cultural trauma, and others are not. Needless to say, this approach to cultural trauma is a constructivist view of social relations, inscribing them in discourse and material conditions. In this view, cultural acts of representation and reception are entwined in the formation of traumatic subjectivity. For example, describing the effects of African-American slavery filtered through the generations, Ron Eyerman says there is a 'difference between trauma as it affects individuals and as a cultural process' (1). In the progression from individual trauma to cultural trauma a new historical narrative emerges around the event in question.

Locating trauma in the domain of shared experiences and as enacted through cultural transmission are matters still under consideration and the challenge to the boundaries of individuated bodies and subjects is not always welcome. Some, like Ruth Leys in *Trauma: A Genealogy,* have strenuously queried this trend to applying the term in non-clinical accounts. In addition, there are concerns about the broadness of its application, raising the logical question of when is something painful *not* trauma?[6] Hans Joas worries that 'the notion of cultural trauma can be extended to whole cultures' as though it is an endemic illness (367), but the notion of a 'whole culture' is not essential to the Yale model that subtends Alexander's work. Cultural trauma does not insist that society can be so circumscribed, nor that culture is homogenous. Alexander's emphasis is on collectivities, and I take these to be contingent, historically located groupings which may, for example, be gathered at local, regional, or national levels, or defined in terms of gendered, ethnic or otherwise identified collectives. Wulf Kansteiner would rather critics had not challenged the original clinical definition of trauma being 'outside the range' of usual human experience (213–14); however, as feminists have already argued, by broadening the clinical range of experiences deemed traumatic (that is, *not* outside the range) awareness was raised of traumatic experiences inflected by gender, especially rape and domestic violence.[7] Trauma is not constituted only in terms of unusual, discrete, individual distress; in fact, particular traumas may be defined and maintained by cultural conditions. Further, although the above examples might suggest otherwise, not all cultural traumas come in the wake of intentional acts of injury. In fact, the concept of cultural trauma as it emerges in Alexander's work is of particular value for evaluating social and cultural situations where structural violence is the issue, and neither the victims nor the perpetrators are singular.

My particular interest here is an episode of cultural trauma which has a more limited audience and local geography. The Chamberlain murder trial, also known as 'the dingo case', polarised the Australian community. On 17 August 1980 a nine-week-old baby, Azaria Chamberlain, disappeared from her parents' tent at an Ayers Rock campsite.[8] Her mother was convinced the child had been taken by a dingo seen near the family tent; yet at the time, dingoes were thought of as scavengers not hunters and assumed to be wary of people. Subsequently, after a long and very public police investigation, her mother was charged with murder and sent to trial. In 1982, Lindy Chamberlain was convicted by a jury in the Northern Territory and sentenced to ninety-nine years imprisonment with hard labour in a Darwin prison. Relentless media scrutiny and stigmatisation of Lindy Chamberlain contributed to the miscarriage of justice that saw her incarcerated for three and a half years before her release and the eventual overturning of the conviction and payment of compensation for wrongful imprisonment.

The Chamberlain case is a complex historical scene, too large to revisit here, but a number of book and article publications have addressed its socio-cultural facets in terms of gender, media, popular culture, nationalism and forensic law.[9] Elsewhere, I have raised questions about of the legal and public violence construed by the Chamberlain case; I argue that the pain-delivering medieval underpinnings of modern day law, one of the governing instruments which manage society, gave traumatic resonance to the Chamberlain case.[10] The Chamberlain case illustrates the violence that law does, especially in sentencing and any wrongful imprisonment. Lindy Chamberlain's suffering through the justice system was a legal and hence public trauma because of the institutions involved. However, my interest here is the transformation of this episode of private, individual suffering, and public culpability, into the broader historical dimensions of a cultural trauma.

The model of cultural trauma draws attention to the redefinition of events and interpretation of memories as a process of cultural meaning-making. The emphasis on the role of the cultural carriers (i.e. journalists, academics, politicians, community activists) in this approach to cultural trauma highlights the instrumentality of cultural power across everyday life. The contribution of cultural carriers and national debates in the processing of the Chamberlain case is central to how it is understood and remembered, as I shall demonstrate. Here, I turn to textual evidence of the case's reception as a traumatic event by reading a sample of the Chamberlain Papers (National Library of Australia MS9180): some

20,000 letters from the public to Lindy Chamberlain now held in the National Library.[11]

Life Writing as Witness to Trauma

If, following Alexander's model, the emergence of a cultural trauma requires claim-making, acts of reinterpretation, and evidence of experience, affect, and thought, then archives of life writing must emerge as potentially rich resources. With such an archive, one might account for public perceptions and the genesis of cultural trauma. Letters and diaries, in particular, often provide the accounts of everyday life that historians call primary sources and activists call testimony. They can provide evidence of *collective* experience that takes up and perhaps even overwhelms the originary event in the production of a new narrative. Substantial archives of life writing relating to a particular event become especially valuable in examining the emergence of cultural trauma, and its discursive formations in the public sphere. Its artefacts can enable us to rethink the history of this particular event and its societal impact, by enabling us to re-examine the fragile boundaries between the private and public spheres when personal tragedy becomes a locus of collective experience.

Life writing may well prove to be an important primary source of data on culturally traumatic events, if the Chamberlain Papers are any indication. This archive is an evidence trail, a discourse stream, and reading across its strata enables traumatic incoherence to divulge a telling narrative. The archive was formed from the thousands upon thousands of cards, letters, and requests sent to Lindy Chamberlain over the years. This correspondence tended to peak around the legal episodes she was involved in: inquests, the trial, appeals, and her final release, as well as anniversaries of family significance. She continued to save these items, and another peak in the correspondence followed the release of her autobiography, *Through My Eyes*, in 1990. This collection was purchased by the NLA in the mid-1990s, and most of it is available to the public.

What are the implications of the fact that Lindy Chamberlain is the subject of the second largest personal file in the NLA, its contents ranging from Azaria's hospital name swatch to the long letter from a former detective apologising for his prejudice? Most clearly, the 20,000 items in the NLA's Chamberlain Papers provide extraordinary material evidence that Lindy Chamberlain experienced a groundswell of support from the public, who literally rallied to her cause, wrote tens of thousands of letters, and successfully petitioned for a Royal Commission (an independent judicial inquiry) into her conviction. Most of the correspondence is one way; as Lindy Chamberlain-Creighton explains in her autobiography, she and her family relied on a mass-mailed newsletter to keep her in touch with her many supporters. However, the archive does bear the imprint of Lindy Chamberlain-Creighton herself—through her marginalia, her cataloguing, her occasional responses, and the closed files. They also show a nation dealing with an event which, for a number of intersecting reasons, they found traumatic.

I therefore read these letters as traumatic residue, or traumata, evidence of a many layered and widely distributed cultural trauma, and signs of collective as well as individual grief. These letters to Lindy Chamberlain—before, during and after her trial, conviction and incarceration—demonstrate the public's empathy for her suffering, and that they felt traumatised in witnessing her persecution. In particular, they reflect on personal loss, courageous suffering, issues of national identity and a failing justice system. The letters show that while the case was mediated by cultural carriers in a variety of ways (for instance, hostility, vilification, prosecution, penalty), the letter-writers established an intimate relationship with Lindy Chamberlain mainly based on notions of her suffering; these accentuated particularly the injustice of her conviction, and her grief as a mother, for the disappearance and death of daughter Azaria, the removal of newborn Kahlia Chamberlain from her care, and the lengthy separation from her two sons Reagan and Aidan Chamberlain due to wrongful imprisonment.

The letters are evidence of the emergence, adoption and circulation of the language of trauma in relation to the Chamberlains' experience. Firstly, the traumatic vicissitudes of Lindy Chamberlain's experience were not opaque to the letter writing public. The letter-writers are persuasive in their assessment of just what constituted this trauma. Letter-writers repeatedly stated that they regarded Lindy Chamberlain as a subject of traumatic circumstances: when her child is taken by a dingo, when she is victimised by the media, when she has to endure wrongful conviction and imprisonment, and when she is forcibly separated from her husband and surviving young children. They did this without ambivalence:

> you have been treated very unjustly and very cruelly, both by the legal system & the media, & that I think you should not be in goal now & never should have been.[12]

> Although we have never met I hurt for you [. . .][13]

Like her grieving face at trial, and her terribly thin appearance when released from prison, they observe in these signs the presence of 'trauma'.[14]

But in addition to this, the Library's collection presents what might be called, to borrow a phrase, an 'archive of feelings', that articulates these events as traumatic *to the collective*.[15] This set of life writings documents a communal sense of injury; the community describes their experience of witnessing the case, and of being collectively responsible to a miscarriage of justice, as traumatic. The letters form a discursive public and together they collect the Chamberlain case within the range of traumatic experience. The letters are handwritten, using scratchy biro and sometimes coloured pencil, and may at first seem unlikely acknowledgements of persecution and pain compared to a clinical definition, or a formal apology from the state. But the letter-writers took up a position of witnessing, and they grieved with the Chamberlains. For instance, when Lindy Chamberlain's baby born just after sentencing was removed by the state, many describe how they wept at the news:

> Dear Mrs Chamberlain, I have been going to write for some time to express my deep sympathy for the treatment you have received. Today topped it off when I heard you could not keep your baby. I am shedding tears for you [...].[16]

> [...] I have wept many times for you and my heart breaks at the thought of your coming separation from your new little baby.[17]

Amongst its many facets, this cultural trauma needs to be understood in terms of how maternity was figured. In response to the forced separation of Lindy Chamberlain and her child, some correspondents made offers to foster baby Kahlia, in a gesture of communality with maternal responsibilities.

In addition, they relayed episodes of private trauma as points of empathy with the Chamberlain's public experience.[18] Here we see signs of compassionate identification, exemplified by the common refrain, 'I often imagine what it is like to be in your place'. Compassionate identification is a work of imagination, and a hope expressed that the letter can make a difference. In many cases, especially in connection with the activities of the support groups, writing letters did make a material difference. They may have felt 'sorry' and 'ashamed' at how she was treated and the situation they found themselves in, as mediatised witnesses.[19] However, this was not a position of passivity, so much as one of affective agency. The articulation of a cultural trauma would not be possible without this compassionate identification, this taking on of another's pain and suffering. Through the function of witnessing, atomised experiences can be re-cast as social knowledge, as part of the communal storehouse of knowledge. It is basic to the movement of events from individual to collective ownership, and the collective's association of those events with a particular set of feelings. In the archive of letters, then, we can discern the accretion of a cultural trauma witnessed, felt, and expressed, then rendered in a discursive formation.

Many of the letter-writers articulated Lindy Chamberlain's position as one of courageous agency. Her strength, her resolute defence of her innocence, her stoic sanity when they took her baby daughter away from her, were qualities much admired by many of the letter-writers:

> I used to write to you when you were in prison and have always believed in you. To me, you are a heroic woman and a shining example to us all of courage and faith. How you have weathered all the storms thrown at you I will never know there must be a purpose in it all & you must be a very special person to have been chosen in this way. So much strength in the face of so much pain & suffering.[20]

That many saw Lindy Chamberlain as a martyr, as chosen by God's will for a purpose, as special to God, and likened her ordeal to 'Christ suffering on the Cross',[21] will come as no surprise, since the case was always overshadowed by the intense interest of the media in her religious beliefs. Connected with this, is critical commentators' description of the case as a witchunt.[22] Thus, there is a strongly Christian element in the letters archive; yet, others asserted their secularity and felt it important, in stating their support for Lindy Chamberlain, to distinguish themselves as 'not of' the Chamberlain's religion.[23] With this move, they claimed a civic connection. They too found an agency in the act of witnessing, with or without its religious undertones.

Life Writing as Counter-Narrative

There is no question that the loss of Azaria Chamberlain was a personal disaster for Lindy Chamberlain and the Chamberlain family; and the murder trial and media persecution delivered an individual experience of trauma to Lindy Chamberlain and her children. Yet, it is the significance of the events for the Australian public that I wish to highlight, via the evidence of the letters. This case was divisive, and the contestation of meanings around the events is recorded in the letters. In them, the issues, the extremes of emotion, and the sheer number of correspondents suggests an episode of cultural trauma. Indeed, the Chamberlain case's representation across so many cultural domains is typical of the process that Alexander attributes to cultural trauma: the trauma is embodied and replayed in eight different judicial processes, in a library archive of staggering proportions, in National Museum exhibits, in cinema and television, and in a number of works of art and literature. These mediums are discursive horizons for the articulation of social concerns, and the Chamberlain case precipitated an array of television shows, paintings, books, magazine articles, movies, pop songs, jokes and cartoons, and poems—as well as the astonishing 20,000 items now held at the NLA. In Alexander's terms, these cultural productions are the work of cultural carriers, and the sites in which a revised historical narrative may emerge. Debate about the social impact of an event, claims for and against its wounding nature, a contestation of interpretation and of feeling, exemplifies a working through of the past for reasons that may not be fully apparent at the time. The proliferation of cultural product around the Chamberlain case offers a wide-ranging and diverse uptake of elements of the story, and is highly suggestive in terms of genre, medium, and institutional location.

Amongst these, letter writing presents an interesting case: whilst firmly ensconced within the domain of writing, is not an elite domain—historically it is seen as domestic, or leisurely, and indeed, feminine and private. But these letters were acquired by the Library at a time when it was becoming more acknowledged, especially in literary studies, that acts of private letter and diary writing are significant in terms of social and cultural practice.[24] Whilst the NLA remains discreet about what it paid for the Chamberlain Papers, it appears that the Library estimated the value of the Chamberlain collection not only for its research potential but also its 'symbolic' significance and as a source of 'collective memory'[25] in other words, for somewhat intangible cultural values.

We can also think of these cultural productions as signalling the fragmented and ongoing *reception* of traumatic events that began at Ayers Rock in 1980, for each has their own audiences. However often the story of the Chamberlain case is retold, its insistent return suggests a history still to be possessed by its people. This, too, is a sign of trauma: the failure to achieve resolution or catharsis. Clearly the case indicates unfinished business in the collective, and the letter-writers amplify the perception that the public persecution of Lindy Chamberlain was a traumatic experience for which Australian citizens bore a collective responsibility.

Whilst in formal processes of historical revision and reconciliation an event may be largely circumscribed by official doctrine, less obvious (and usually less accessible) are those instances where the process of coming to terms with a traumatic event is conducted privately, and by a large number of people. And, if the collection of letters is any indication, this processing is ongoing. As the majority of the letters are sympathetic to Lindy Chamberlain and her family, these letters resist the court and media assertions of Chamberlain's guilt, and they call into question the mediatised view that the public was largely against her.[26] The strongest, most consistent theme across all of the letters is Lindy Chamberlain's innocence of the crime for which she is at first suspected, then tried, convicted and imprisoned for. This leads me to read the letter-writers as presenting a community of dissent. However, unlike cultural carriers positioned to publicly comment on the case by means of their profession or social standing, the letter-writers tend to make their claims with reference to feeling a commonality with Lindy Chamberlain or by indexing loose socio-cultural networks (Australians, mothers, the legal fraternity, Christians, immigrants). Those letters in the Chamberlain Papers which make intertextual references to family, friends, and local religious groups demonstrate this tendency, and so too do the frequent refrain of the letters to Lindy Chamberlain: 'we have never met but . . .' What these letters reveal is a constituency formed around the reception of this event. It is a relationship that articulates the phenomenon of celebrity and the interpersonal aspect of handwritten letters into a discursive formation of the public.

The letters therefore come to embody an oppositional or counter-narrative of unheralded voices; that is, a discursive resistance to the predominant vilification of Chamberlain. In fact, the letters must be seen as the cultural carriers and their words as issuing the counter-narrative. The momentum for counter-narrative is underpinned by the letters' common tropes of suffering, overwhelming emotion, and loss. That the Chamberlain case, in terms of its originary trauma in the death of Azaria, and its elements of persecution, was a tragedy is without doubt. But the archive suggests that the case meant more to people than this individuated injury. The letter-writers enunciated their concerns without either hesitation or confusion, and their collective weight is inescapable: Chamberlain was innocent, a gross miscarriage of justice had occurred, the nation was sullied by a 'shameful' verdict.[27] Whilst the police and the media used their professional positions to speak from, many of the letter-writers simply understood themselves to be writing as 'public citizens' in defence of national standards of justice.[28] They describe the Chamberlain case as a 'violation of civil rights'.[29] Perceptions of injustice would appear to have weighed heavily on the letter-writers; they viewed the trial as an injury to themselves and their cultural traditions:

> I am one of the many people who are heart-broken and ashamed because of the cruelty and injustice you have suffered. We are proud of you and your family and the courage you have shown [...] there are thousands who know as I do that you are innocent.[30]

> The demise of the importance of human testimony under Christian oath in favour of the trial by microscope and media frightened a lot of Australians. And angered them, too.[31]

Letter-writers perceived the Chamberlain case as an 'outrage'[32] and a 'horror',[33] a miscarriage of justice that threatened all Australians. In one letter to the editor of the *Sydney Morning Herald* newspaper, the accusation against state forces was put in blunt terms:

> I don't see why her children have to suffer [... and] this family has to suffer by the stupidity of the NT Government [...] Would the SMH consider opening an appeal for the Chamberlains so as to shame that bunch of beer sodden bureaucrats and their police force to come to their senses [...]?[34]

This desire to restore justice is also apparent in the thousands of signatures submitted by the Chamberlain Support Groups on formal petitions (see Young). As one of the letter-writers points out, over time, people found the Chamberlain case and Lindy Chamberlain's imprisonment to be a matter of 'conscience'.[35] The sense of civic responsibility that this appeal to conscience invokes is typical of witnessing and its aspirations to prevent the repetition of wrongs. In their private communications to Lindy Chamberlain, it is evident that the miscarriage of justice was taken to reflect poorly on the nation, and the divisive effects of the case demonstrated emerging rifts in a hegemonic image of Australia as the place of 'a fair go'.[36] The divisive aspects of the Chamberlain case, its rupture of hegemony, are an indication of deeply contested histories in social narratives of nation in Australia.

A Stolen Child

The 1990s in Australia was a period in which debates on globalisation, multiculturalism and difference were vigorously addressed as topics of national interest. This culminated in the federally legislated and funded, ten-year social project of the Council for Aboriginal Reconciliation, 1991–2000. Most importantly, in Australia as elsewhere, *discourses* of reconciliation were increasingly used, whether or not the practices produced actual change. Reconciliation was signified as a 'renewal of the nation' (Australian Reconciliation Convention): in other words, a re-imagining of Australian identity. It was to encompass issues of race relations, nationhood, power, Australian space, narrative, history and identity, and it effected a massive critique of white Australia. The period saw public intellectuals intervene in 'the stolen generations issue as brought to light by the *Bringing Them Home* report (from 1997); the subsequent refusal of [Prime Minister] Howard to apologise to Indigenous Australians; the mounting debate over reconciliation; and most recently the debate over genocide and massacres'.[37] In the formulation of individual trauma into cultural trauma around the Chamberlain case we can see how this episode intersected with, and perhaps was a testing ground for, critical issues of Australian identity foregrounded in the 1990s.

It is possible that the impact of the Chamberlain case upon ideas of the nation was germinal to the sea change in national identity that was to follow in Australia's path to Reconciliation. Indeed, the letters evince a number of issues over which the later struggle for Australian identity was to take place: relationships to the land, to Indigenous people and their knowledge, and to the legitimacy of aspects of white culture such as the authority of the state, police, judiciary, media and science. To conceive of it this way, it is necessary to move beyond reading the Chamberlain case as just another episode of legal bungling; rather, what people felt they were witnessing was an historic wrong.[38] The reluctance of the state to acknowledge that wrong uncannily parallels the problem that the Australian state has had with acknowledging the dispossession of its indigenous people of their children. For this reason, I suggest that the traumatic impact of the Chamberlain case was amplified by the then-unspoken crime of the 'Stolen Generations'—those Aboriginal children forcibly removed from their mothers by various Australian agencies, up to at least 1969—that gained immense pubic attention with the publication of an inquiry into the history of these removals.[39]

What are the correlations between the forced separation of Indigenous Australian children from their families and the Chamberlain case? How could the then-hidden trauma of the Stolen Generations have been a backdrop to the disappearance and death of Azaria? The Stolen Generations are so patently an historic and culture-wide event of trauma,[40] that although the term Stolen Generations did not have meaning until more than a decade later, the link that I posit between the two episodes of public debate is neither anachronistic nor unlikely. For the Stolen Generations were taken by the state from their mothers many years *before* Azaria Chamberlain was taken from her tent by a predator, and this was an unacknowledged trauma up until the decade *following* the resolution of the Chamberlain case. Thus, the Chamberlain case touched on an already deep and emotive wound that lay unexposed—one that had, at the time, little public voice. Lindy Chamberlain's experience of loss appears to have tapped directly into both real and imagined traumas of the Australian settler past.[41] The cases are not equal, but I suspect that the treatment of one resonated with the denial of the other. In retrospect, the excesses of anxiety, grief and guilt in the Australian public around the Chamberlain case are made more explicable when read against a nation denying its responsibility for a terrible history of stolen children.

Some twenty-two years after Azaria's disappearance, here is how Kay Schaffer describes the national, traumatic impact of the Stolen Generations:

> Genocide, Trauma, Guilt, Shame, Willful Forgetting, Denial. Before the release of *Bringing Them Home: Report of the Forced Separation of Aboriginal Children from their Families* (1997) these words were not part of the Australian lexicon. Now they are. Before the release of the report these terms resonated with popular understandings of the horrors of the German Holocaust. They had no relevance for Australia. Or so we thought [...]. (1)

It is the relevance of these terms to Australian identity that the public reactions to the Chamberlain case seem to prefigure. I find the parallels inescapable, and they suggest that the cultural trauma that emerged around this miscarriage of justice that featured the grieving mother of a baby taken in the desert, and a subsequent forced separation from her other children, drew upon a deeply embedded trauma that would finally be acknowledged through the public reporting of the Stolen Generations. That is, the unspoken trauma of the Stolen Generations seems to have created a resonance chamber in which elements of the disappearance of Azaria and the Chamberlain trial were remade and amplified. The social and cultural context which generated traumatic responses to the Chamberlain case included the genocide of Indigenous Australians, through the transfer of their children.[42]

Of course, the cases are not parallel in a number of key respects: the Stolen Generations are an episode of genocide, the death of Azaria Chamberlain was not; the persecution of Lindy Chamberlain, however atrocious, differs from the intent behind acts of genocide; and the politics of race discrimination is a crucial factor in the Stolen Generations that had minimal bearing on how Lindy Chamberlain was treated.[43] Further, it is possible to imagine the Chamberlain case as being a cultural trauma without drawing on its connections with any other particular historical wrong. But that would be to massively decontextualise it from its Australian base. For the theme of dispossession has more general applications. The Chamberlain case took place in a settler society, a land of dispossessed peoples, not all of whom were indigenes (see Carter *Dispossession*). Migrant and Indigenous populations often draw on representations of themselves being dispossessed peoples, albeit this dispossession has been experienced very differently. In a figurative, if not literal sense, Lindy Chamberlain variously represented the sufferings of the dispossessed: loss of family, of liberty, financial struggle, disenfranchisement, and a destruction of self. This figure emerged in a land of dispossessed peoples; perhaps it is not surprising that many identified with Lindy Chamberlain's experience as a victim of state injustice and cultural prejudices. Perhaps in communicating with Lindy Chamberlain, people from the margins sought both to identify and be heard. Yet, this is rather different from saying that Lindy Chamberlain herself was a compelling figure of cultural difference—as a white, middle-class, Christian housewife and mother, she was hardly an illustration of cultural difference. Yet her status as a coastal dweller, her persistent claims that a dingo took her baby, and the fact that she did not perform her grief and mourning in public, were remarked as a refusal of Australia's dominant white, masculinist, middle-class culture which insisted on particular behaviours from its women and adherence to idealised notions of the outback.[44]

Just as the archive of letters reveals a long history of support for the Chamberlains, they also move across a series of different moments in the unfolding events, and changes of heart. These changes are shaped by the specific ongoing developments in the case, as well as reflecting shifting cultural values. A sense of this emerges in the letters to Lindy Chamberlain. As reconciliation around sites of historical trauma became normal, these emerging public practices inflected and rendered possible a changing public memory of Lindy Chamberlain. This offers another important reading from the letters, this time of the apologies sent to Lindy Chamberlain by those who had a change of heart. These letters are read as acts of reconciliation. The letters of apology started arriving and: 'many, many are focussed on their guilt at believing her guilty' (Howe, personal correspondence). Apology and regret are strong themes across the letters. The letters reveal that more than a few of the Australian public recognised their own culpability in Lindy Chamberlain's persecution. Whilst they may have directed Lindy Chamberlain to 'come to terms with' her own grief, they also marked a need of the nation to say sorry:

> I am very pleased to have the opportunity to say 'sorry' for having thought that you were guilty of the death of your baby girl, Azaria. [...] How cruel we all were, sorry is not good enough. We can only try to let you live in peace & hang our heads in shame at the pain you have gone through.[45]

The letters put a mirror to the witnesses' shame, and the violence of beliefs, as many regret their vehement opposition to Lindy Chamberlain's innocence. They wrote to Lindy to beg her apology for their doubting of her, and the message this gives us is of a cultural movement towards working through.

This echoes Alexander's model of cultural trauma in which the generating of public memory is an ongoing, and not necessarily immediate, process that is shaped by social change. These cultural processes produce historical accounts that compete with, and sometimes displace each other, over time. The meaning of the past in the present is not self-evident, it emerges from contestation, and any emerging formations of cultural trauma are part of the process. Confronting an unjust past is a powerful strategy in refusing its repetition. Michael Humphrey suggests that, in remembering persecution, such pain becomes a medium through which historical wrongs can be represented to the community (106). This can be seen in some episodes of mass atrocity followed by socially orchestrated processes of remembrance and reconciliation, for example, the public hearings for the Republic of South Africa Truth and Reconciliation Commissions. In these processes, what was unspeakable is spoken, what was invisible is publicised, and social differences are recognised and perhaps reconciled through these kinds of discursive shifts. In the Australian context, witnessing the Chamberlain case was perhaps one way, however indirectly, of recognising a painful past and reinvigorating the public sphere with concerns about the state's powers of dispossession.

Conclusion

Traumatic repetition is about the inability to conclude an aspect of history, an inability which brokers a traumatic relationship. In her autobiography, Lindy Chamberlain expressed it this way: 'I cannot begin to count the personal cost of the last ten years. The total effects on the lives of myself and my family are permanent and far-reaching' (xiii). These effects have their longevity, I argue, because they are traumatic within the framework of the individual life histories of Lindy and her family (as she attests here) and also because of the more extended frameworks of cultural trauma; in both contexts they have the far reaching and repetitive structure of trauma. Once the Chamberlain case is perceived as a traumatically *structuring* event, the various cultural productions that it precipitated (paintings, poetry, opera, television drama, Hollywood feature film) appear like the dreamwork of trauma victims, repetitively returning to un-integrated events. Alexander would identify this as the work of cultural carriers, both identifying and transmitting cultural trauma. A traumatic ambivalence about the event—remembered but not fully grasped—gives it a haunting afterlife in the culture.

By focusing on these letters as a discursive formation of the public, I show that even the most humble of handwritten letters can inform the public sphere; that life writing can at times take on larger causes; and that it has a commemorative function. These are the cultural productions that might signal the development of a new narrative and the reshaping of cultural memory. It is through these ongoing representations that recognition of the significance of the Chamberlain case as cultural trauma is advanced. Trauma experienced by the few, but represented to the whole, can become incorporated into the dominant viewpoint as a cultural trauma. Academics have a role to play in this process, as do writers, television producers and others involved in communicating important issues. It would appear that Lindy Chamberlain has by now been recuperated into the mythos of nation in a positive sense, as a figure of courage in the face of societal prejudice and institutional wrongs. The Chamberlain case thus remains alive in shaping the Australian public conscience. And, by reading together what seem to be very different traumas of the recent past—the Chamberlain case and the Stolen Generations—we are in a position to narrate what circulates as cultural trauma in the life of the Australian nation.

Notes

[1] See Connerton for further discussion of the ways in which memory is physically embodied.

[2] To use Jeffrey Alexander's term.

[3] For example, see Terry Maroney; Olga Tsoudis and Lynn Smith-Lovin; Heather Strang and John Braithwaite.

[4] For example, see Wolfgang Schivelbusch; Michael Humphrey; Gitta Sereny; Antonius Robben and Marcel Suarez-Orozco.

[5] This is a paraphrased version.

[6] See Hans Joas; Wulf Kansteiner.

[7] See Laura Brown; Maria Root.

[8] Since being returned to its traditional Aboriginal custodians, the site formerly known as Ayers Rock is properly named Uluru–Kata Tjuta National Park.

[9] See Kerryn Goldsworthy; Adrian Howe; Noel Sanders; Julie Marcus; Trevor Morling; John Bryson.

[10] See Deborah Staines.

[11] Separately, the Library also maintains several other collections related to the case: Norman Young's research papers from his book on the activities of the various Chamberlain support groups; papers from prominent Chamberlain supporters such as the Boyd family; and of course the Neville Dawson oil portraits of Lindy Chamberlain and the prosecution's Ian Barker QC. Further references to the Library herein abbreviated as NLA.

[12] Except where indicated with referencing, the use of quotation marks (' ') in the following text indicates direct citations from the Chamberlain letters. I have quoted only from directly cited sources, and withheld the personal details of the letter-writers. However, an exact record of all sources (name, date, box number) is retained by the author. Copyright is formally held by the individual letter-writers.

[13] New South Wales (NSW), 1984.

[14] Multiple citations. No location, 1982; NSW, 1988; WA, 1991; Queensland (QLD), 1991; New Zealand (NZ), undated.

[15] To borrow Ann Cvetkovich's term.

[16] WA, 1982.
[17] NSW, 1982.
[18] These stories too might be considered traumatic residue (traumata) in their own right. Many shared tales of loss, grief and failure with Lindy Chamberlain and these are conveyed to readers of the archive. They are carried into history by their location within the pubic archive. Unfortunately, a study of this aspect of the archive is beyond the scope of this article.
[19] QLD, undated; Victoria (VIC) 1984.
[20] NZ, 1992.
[21] No location, undated.
[22] See Paul Toohey; A. N. Maiden.
[23] WA, 1984.
[24] See David Barton and Nigel Hall.
[25] See Adrian Cunningham.
[26] A common question about the archives is whether abusive or critical letters were retained. Lindy Chamberlain-Creighton herself created a singular file entitled 'Nut letters' for those she found most extreme, and these are held within the Collection. In addition, scattered throughout the archive are letters from people with obviously mixed feelings about the case; it is up to the reader to evaluate the significance of these. It does not appear that Lindy Chamberlain-Creighton weeded out a percentage of the material for any particular reason, other than the small number of closed files which are scheduled for future release. It is more likely that these represent private family matters than accusatory letters from strangers.
[27] NSW, undated; South Australia (SA), undated.
[28] Northern Territory (NT), 1985.
[29] VIC, 1992.
[30] NSW, 1985.
[31] NSW, 1986.
[32] WA, 1984; NSW, 1982.
[33] SA, undated; NSW, 1982; QLD 1991.
[34] NSW, 1989.
[35] SA, 1991.
[36] NSW, 1983.
[37] See David Carter; Stuart Macintyre.
[38] Lindy Chamberlain-Creighton is still waiting on a death certificate that declares that her daughter died of dingo attack. The Northern Territory Government has not offered a formal apology for the Territory's treatment of the Chamberlains. The fact that this wrong still has not been entirely righted, twenty-five years later, is an indication of what was placed at stake by Lindy Chamberlain's claim that an Australian dingo killed Azaria.
[39] See Human Rights and Equal Opportunity Commission.
[40] See Roseanne Kennedy.
[41] In addition, the missing child was an already-iconic figure in Australian culture (see Pierce). It recurs throughout Australian literature, art and film as a cipher for the fragility of Australian settlement. It represents the indigenous bush as a fearful threat to the cohesion of the family life outside of settled, city spaces.
[42] Colin Tatz summarises the report's case for genocide thus: 'The National Inquiry reported in April 1997. Of the 118 official investigations—judicial inquiries, parliamentary committee reports and royal commissions—into aspects of Aboriginal affairs this century, this is by far the starkest and strongest indictment, concluding that Australia has knowingly committed genocide through the forcible transfer of children, as a matter of official policy, not just yesteryear but as recently as the 1970s. A finding of genocide was presented: the essence of the crime, it was stated,

was acting with the intention of destroying the group, not the extent to which that intention was achieved. The forcible removals were intended to "absorb," "merge," "assimilate" the children so that Aborigines as a distinct group would disappear' (1–40).

[43] See Phillipa Sawyer.

[44] Jocelyn Scutt; Julie Marcus.

[45] NSW, 2000.

References

Alexander, Jeffrey C. 'Toward a Theory of Cultural Trauma.' *Cultural Trauma and Collective Identity*. Ed. Jeffrey Alexander, et al. Berkeley: U of California P, 2004. 1–30.

Australian Reconciliation Convention. *The Path to Reconciliation: Renewal of the Nation*. ACT: Australian Government Publishing Service, 1997.

Barton, David, and Nigel Hall, eds. *Letter Writing as a Social Practice*. Philadelphia, PA: Benjamins Publishing, 1999.

Brown, Laura S. 'Not Outside the Range: One Feminist Perspective on Psychic Trauma.' *Trauma: Explorations in Memory*. Ed. Cathy Caruth. Baltimore, MD: Johns Hopkins UP, 1995. 100–12.

Bryson, John. *Evil Angels*. Ringwood, Victoria: Penguin, 1986.

Carter, David. *Dispossession, Dreams and Diversity: Issues in Australian Studies*. Frenchs Forest, NSW: Pearson Longman, 2006.

———. 'Public Intellectuals, Book Culture and Civil Society.' *Australian Humanities Review* Dec.–Feb. (2001–02): n.p.

Chamberlain, Lindy. *Through My Eyes: An Autobiography*. Port Melbourne: William Heinmann Australia, 1990.

Connerton, Paul. *How Societies Remember*. Cambridge: Cambridge UP, 1989.

Cunningham, Adrian. 'Icons, Symbolism and Recordkeeping: The Lindy Chamberlain and Eddie Mabo Papers in the National Library of Australia.' *Australian Academic and Research Libraries* 28.2 (1997): 103–10.

Cvetkovich, Ann. *An Archive of Feelings: Trauma, Sexuality, and Lesbian Public Cultures*. Durham, NC: Duke UP, 2003.

Eyerman, Ron. *Cultural Trauma: Slavery and the Formation of African-American Identity*. Cambridge: Cambridge UP, 2002.

Goldsworthy, Kerryn. 'Martyr to Her Sex.' *Oxford Book of Australian Essays*. Oxford: OUP, 1997. 258–62.

Howe. Personal interview.

Howe, Adrian. 'Chamberlain Revisited: The Case Against the Media.' *Gender, Crime and Feminism*. Ed. Ngaire Naffine. Aldershot, England: Dartmouth, 1995. 175–81.

———. 'Imagining Evidence, Fictioning Truth—Revisiting (Courtesy of OJ Simpson) Expert Evidence in the Chamberlain Case.' *Law Text Culture* 3 (1997): 83–106.

Human Rights and Equal Opportunity Commission. *Bringing Them Home: Report of the National Inquiry into the Separation of Aboriginal and Torres Strait Islander Children from their Families*. Sydney, Australia: Human Rights and Equal Opportunity Commission, 1997.

Humphrey, Michael. *The Politics of Atrocity and Reconciliation: From Terror to Trauma*. London: Routledge, 2002.

Joas, Hans. 'Cultural Trauma? On the Most Recent Turn in Jeffrey Alexander's Cultural Sociology.' *European Journal of Social Theory* 8 (2005): 365–74.

Kansteiner, Wulf. 'Genealogy of a Category Mistake: A Critical Intellectual History of the Cultural Trauma Metaphor.' *Rethinking History* 8.2 (2004): 193–221.

Kennedy, Roseanne. 'Stolen Generations Testimony: Trauma, Historiography, and the Question of Truth.' *Aboriginal History* 25 (2002): 116–31.

Leys, Ruth. *Trauma: A Genealogy.* Chicago: U of Chicago P, 2000.

Macintyre, Stuart. *A Concise History of Australia.* Melbourne: Cambridge UP, 1999.

Maiden, A. N. 'Witchunt: How the Chamberlain Case Touched a Nation's Inner Fears.' *Time Australia* 15 June 1987: 32–35.

Marcus, Julie. 'Prisoner of Discourse: The Dingo, the Dog and the Baby.' *Anthropology Today* 5.3 (1989): 15–19.

Maroney, Terry. 'Law and Emotion: A Proposed Taxonomy of an Emerging Field.' *Law and Human Behaviour* 30.2 (2006): 119–42.

Morling, Trevor. *Report of the Commissioner the Hon. Mr. Justice T.R. Morling.* Darwin: Government Printer, 1987.

National Library of Australia. MS9180. Canberra.

Pierce, Peter. *The Country of Lost Children: An Australian Anxiety.* Cambridge: Cambridge UP, 1999.

Robben, Antonius C. G. M., and Marcelo M. Suarez-Orozco, eds. *Cultures Under Siege: Collective Violence and Trauma.* Cambridge UP, 2000.

Root, Maria P. P. 'Reconstructing the Impact of Trauma on Personality.' *Personality and Psychopathology: Feminist Reappraisals.* Ed. Laura S. Brown and Mary Ballou. New York: Guilford Press, 1992. 229–66.

Sanders, Noel. 'Azaria Chamberlain and Popular Culture.' *Australian Cultural Studies: A Reader.* Ed. John Frow and Meaghan Morris. St Leonards, NSW: Allen & Unwin, 1993. 86–101.

Sawyer, Phillipa. 'Naming Whiteness: An Inquiry into Lindy Chamberlain's *Through My Eyes* and Australian Nationalist Discourses.' *Law Text Culture* 3 (1997): 107–23.

Schaffer, Kay. 'Getting over the Genocide Question: Australia and the Stolen Generations Debates.' *Borderlands e-journal* 1.2 (2002): 1–5.

Schivelbusch, Wolfgang. *The Culture of Defeat: On National Trauma, Mourning, and Recovery.* Trans. Jefferson Chase. New York: Metropolitan Books, 2003.

Scutt, Jocelyn. 'Schemers, Dragons and Witches: Criminal "Justice" and the Fair Sex.' *Stereotypes of Women in Power: Historical Perspectives and Revisionist Views.* New York: Greenwood Press, 1992. 181–208.

Sereny, Gitta. *The German Trauma: Experiences and Reflections, 1938–2000.* London: Allen Lane, 2000.

Smelser, Neil J. 'Psychological Trauma and Cultural Trauma.' *Cultural Trauma and Collective Identity.* Ed. Jeffrey Alexander et al. Berkeley: University of California Press, 2004. 31–59.

Staines, Deborah. 'A Legal Trauma, a Public Trauma: Lindy Chamberlain and the Chamberlain Case.' *Studies in Law, Politics, and Society* 38 (2006): 153–72.

Strang, Heather, and John Braithwaite. *Restorative Justice and Civil Society.* Cambridge: Cambridge UP, 2001.

Tatz, Colin. Genocide in Australia. An AIATSIS Research Discussion Paper, 8. Canberra: Australian Institute of Aboriginal and Torres Strait Islander Studies, 1999, 1–40.

Toohey, Paul. 'Witch Hunt.' *The Australian (Magazine)* 15–16 July 2000: 16–23.

Tsoudis, Olga, and Lynn Smith-Lovin. 'How Bad Was It? The Effects of Victim and Perpetrator Emotion on Responses to Criminal Court Vignettes.' *Social Forces* 77.2 (1998): 695–722.

Young, Norman. *Innocence Regained: The Fight to Free Lindy Chamberlain.* Annandale, NSW: Federation P, 1989.

Vulnerable Children, Disposable Mothers: Holocaust and Stolen Generations Memoirs of Childhood

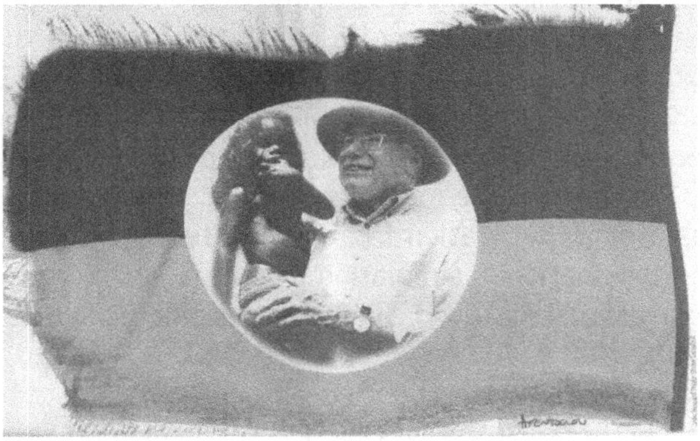

Rosanne Kennedy

Reading Trauma through an Antipodean Lens

Writing about Holocaust testimony, French historian Annette Wieviorka observes that the 1997 trial of Maurice Papon, the last significant war crimes trial in France, marked the delegation of witnessing to a new generation: children who were hidden during the war (145). Esther Fogiel 'mesmerized the audience' with her testimony of the horrific abuse she suffered, including rape, forced labour and psychological abuse, at the hands of a violent couple in whose care her parents had left her, as an eight-year old, before they were deported (146). While insisting that Fogiel is 'an extreme case', Wieviorka observes that 'her sufferings, even her suicide attempt, are echoed' in the experiences of many hidden children who are now expressing themselves (148). Memoirs by hidden children, whom Susan Sulieman describes as the '1.5 generation', extend the cultural memory of the Holocaust. They bring into discourse the legacy of this traumatic past on children whose lives were massively disrupted by persecution and separation from their parents, and who lived in fear of deportation, death and the loss of family (Pine 375). Today these memoirs of Holocaust childhoods circulate alongside narratives of child separation from very different historical and cultural contexts. Their transnational circulation invites a comparative reading that explores how tropes of maternal and child relations emerge in these narratives of traumatic memory.

Sarah Kofman's memoir, *Rue Ordener, Rue Labat*, is an unusual example of 'the hidden child' genre, in part because she was hidden with her mother. A highly regarded French feminist philosopher, Kofman begins her elegantly sparse memoir with her father's arrest in Paris, during the infamous round-up of Jews on July 16, 1942.[1] A rabbi of a small synagogue, he was sent to Drancy and later deported to Auschwitz. After the war, his family was told that he had been brutally beaten and buried alive for praying on the Sabbath rather than working. While the ghost of her father haunts the memoir, the emotional core centres on the eighteen months she and her mother spent in hiding in a small apartment with Meme, a Christian woman 'who loves children' (31). Kofman represents Meme as a captivating but predatory woman who uses the intimate domestic circumstances to lure Sarah away from her mother and Judaism. The strong attachment Sarah forms with Meme results in her estrangement from her mother, which remains an unresolved trauma throughout her life. Rather than echo Fogiel's testimony of childhood innocence and adult tyranny, Kofman's memoir introduces a less familiar and troubling narrative of seduction, betrayal and petty cruelty. Although she was only nine years old, and had already suffered irreparable losses, she positions herself as complicit in the betrayal of her mother. Less than a year after she published this memoir, Kofman took her own life.[2] Her suicide is a potent reminder that bearing witness to trauma does not necessarily aid survival, as the late psychoanalyst Dori Laub had hoped.[3]

Of course, the significance of *Rue Ordener, Rue Labat*, which was published in France in 1994, the year of Paul Trouvier's trial for war crimes, differs depending upon when, where and by whom it is read. In France, Kofman's autobiographical writing coincided with the belated awakening of Jewish memory in the 1980s and 1990s, which historian Henry Russo has dubbed the 'Obsessions' period.[4] During this period the post-war narrative of French resistance was challenged, the role of French police units in arresting and deporting French Jews was exposed, and numerous collaborationist scandals emerged. It was revealed, for instance, that President Mitterand, honoured as a hero in the resistance, was personal friends with Rene Bousquet, chief of Vichy police and organiser of the Vel'd Hiv roundups, whom French Jews were anxious to try for war crimes (Golasan 89). Kofman's memoir of complicity and betrayal echoed the nation's painful confrontation with its hidden past, and exposed the partiality of the heroic narrative offered at Meme's funeral of a woman who 'saved a little Jewish girl during the war' (85).

In Australia, the late 1990s was marked by a long overdue reckoning with the post-colonial legacy of what has become known as the 'Stolen Generations'. In 1996, the Human Rights and Equal Opportunity Commission conducted a landmark National Inquiry into the policies, practices and effects of removing children of mixed Aboriginal and Caucasian descent from their families and communities. The Inquiry travelled around the country collecting testimonies from individuals who had been removed, giving them an opportunity—many for the first time—to tell their stories. Like Esther Fogiel's Holocaust testimony, many Stolen Generations testimonies tell shocking stories of the physical, sexual and emotional abuse of children, and of adulthoods scarred by drug dependency, violence and suicide attempts. Themes of maternal loss and childhood loneliness recur in these testimonies. For example, individuals repeatedly describe being callously removed from their families, and later discovering in their files letters from their grief-stricken mothers, whom they had been told were dead or had abandoned them. In 1997, the Inquiry published its powerful report, *Bringing Them Home*. The cover features a photograph of an Aboriginal woman and child playing a game by a river, framed in silhouette against the sunset. This idealised image of the mother-child relation, associated with nurture, pleasure, intimacy and cultural continuity, intensifies the shock of the violent breaches documented within the text, and signals the value of a maternal trope as a symbolic vehicle for mediating the cultural memory of the Stolen Generations.

Drawing on a discourse of ethical witnessing, *Bringing Them Home* addressed Australians in moral and affective terms, asking them to listen to the testimonies of stolen children with 'open hearts and minds' (Wilson 3). Through this address, the report implicitly positioned the Stolen Generations as victims, and non-Indigenous Australians as belated witnesses to the history of colonisation and child removal. While the report elicited an empathic response from non-Indigenous Australians and generated support for reconciliation, it is important to acknowledge the political and moral limits of empathy. Empathy, when it leads to an unexamined identification with the victim, may distract Australians from recognising our own positions as participants in and beneficiaries of colonisation. [5] As Dominick LaCapra reminds us, in cases of historical injustice, there are often 'divided legacies' —some groups and individuals have been victims while others have benefited, which raises the problem of how to acknowledge and work though 'historical losses in ways that affect different groups differently . . .' (44–45). Rather than acknowledge these divided legacies, the binary of 'victim' and 'belated witness' obscures the range and complexity of subject positions that non-Indigenous and Indigenous Australians occupy in relation to this past.[6] This framing also makes it difficult to acknowledge responses such as denial, ambivalence, and neglect (Kennedy 2004)

In recent years, a number of scholars have been engaged in comparative research on the Holocaust and colonisation in Australia, and have begun to explore these issues.[7] In an insightful essay, Neil Levi contends that a comparative approach can fruitfully throw into relief silences and limits in the discourse of the History Wars in Australia. He argues that a comparative approach to the Holocaust and the Stolen Generations is considered illegitimate by white Australians because we cannot see ourselves as perpetrators of genocide (137–139). Nor, I would add, do we see ourselves as beneficiaries of colonisation. While historians have pioneered comparative approaches to these histories, I suggest that a comparative reading of Stolen Generations and Holocaust memoirs of childhood can generate unique and challenging insights into the complex affective, material and psychological legacies of the assimilation of children across racial and ethnic divides. By bringing Kofman's atypical Holocaust memoir of the seductions and estrangements of assimilation into Antipodean life narrative, I aim to illuminate aspects of Indigenous child removal that have been obscured by the dominant cultural memory of the Stolen Generations.[8]

Kofman's memoir was translated into English in 1996, the year of the National Inquiry.[9] In a discourse that resonates uncannily in Australia, Kofman describes her mother's struggle after the liberation:

> . . . to reclaim me from the woman who wanted to 'steal' me on the pretext that my own mother had more than enough to handle with five other children and wasn't looking after my best interests—which were, according to Meme, not to be raised by my own mother but rather to be brought up by Meme herself (58).

The scenario of Aboriginal children being 'stolen' from their mothers to be raised by white women, alleged to have been in the 'best interests of the child', has figured in Australian cultural narratives of assimilation long before the National Inquiry. For instance, these themes are explored in Charles Chauvel's classic 1955 film *Jedda*, in which a white woman, whose own infant has died, 'rescues' or 'steals' an Aboriginal baby after its mother dies, and raises her as a white child.[10] In *Jedda* white Australians are represented as *participants* in rather than as *belated witnesses* to practices of colonisation and child removal. Mrs McCann, Jedda's adoptive mother, is both a perpetrator and beneficiary of the child's removal, which positions her as complicit in the process of assimilation and cultural loss. Through the blindness that results from her own maternal desire, masked as a 'benevolent intention' to 'improve' Jedda's lot in life, she is implicated in Jedda's estrangement from her culture and her tragic death.

Reflection on the position of the beneficiary has been obscured in Australia by discourses of child protection, and by the sentimental tropes of maternity and childhood that are the preferred readings of narratives of Indigenous child removal and assimilation.[11] Read in this context, Kofman's narrative of theft disavowed as rescue invites reflection on the positions and unacknowledged desires of the beneficiary and the victim.

In this article I read Kofman's memoir in relation to the text and film versions of an important Australian cultural memory of the Stolen Generations. Doris Pilkington's bio-memoir, *Follow the Rabbit-Proof Fence*, published in 1996, tells the story of the removal of her mother Molly, her aunt Daisy and their cousin Gracie from the remote community of Jigalong in the Northern Territory in 1931, when they were aged 14, 11 and 8. Their removal was arranged by A. O. Neville, the Chief Protector of Aborigines in Western Australia. Guided by notions of white superiority and a pseudo-scientific discourse of eugenics, he developed policies to assimilate and 'absorb' Aborigines of mixed descent into the white population and thereby eradicate Aboriginal culture. While Kofman and Pilkington's influences, traditions and styles differ markedly, there are compelling historical reasons for placing their memoirs in dialogue on the subject of maternal tropes in narratives of child separation and assimilation. Pilkington was born in 1936 at Balfour Downs station in Western Australia, two years after Sarah Kofman's birth in Paris. Both were members of groups targeted by the transnational eugenics discourse and policies of the 1930s and 1940s. As a young child, Doris was taken with her mother Molly and her infant sister Annabelle to Moore River Native Settlement, where she remained for the duration of her childhood, after her mother absconded with her sister.[12] Half a world away, Kofman was in hiding from the Gestapo. Both women published memoirs of childhoods disrupted by trauma in the mid-1990s, more than fifty years after the events, exemplifying the insight that 'the belated nature of trauma itself is a transcultural phenomenon' (Brodzki 133).

The Maternal Trope

In one of the few articles to consider the gendering of trauma discourse, psychoanalytic literary critic Claire Kahane reflects upon the frequency with which scenes of anguished separation of mother and child recur in Holocaust literature and film. She argues that '... the profound intimacy between mother and child and its callous violation is a powerful and moving signifier, effectively capturing the perversion of human bonds that was a primary consequence of the Holocaust' (164). As well as signifying trauma and moments of social breakdown, she suggests that writers use the figure of 'the female in pain' because it compels the reader's identification (165). As she reminds us, however, even when scenes of mother and child separation have a historical referent such as the Holocaust or the Stolen Generations, their translation into text '... asks us not merely to experience their painful affect but to question their function within the context of cultural representation and the social effects of their transmission' (165). While Kahane focuses on Holocaust literature, the maternal trope is transcultural in its reach, elastic in its applicability, and discursively mobile. It is regularly used by journalists and filmmakers to mediate unfamiliar or distant events for global audiences, who may lack historical and local knowledge, but can identify with the figure of the suffering woman and child.

In the Australian context, the maternal trope has been ubiquitous in shaping the cultural memory of the Stolen Generations. In the wake of *Bringing Them Home*, which used a mother/child image to frame its findings, the maternal trope has figured in memorials, songs, artwork, films such as *Rabbit-Proof Fence*, and media discourse. Yet, despite its recurrence, scarce attention has been paid to the discursive effects of this gendered trope in shaping the cultural memory of the Stolen Generations. As Marianne Hirsch argues, however, '[a] feminist analysis ... can enhance our understanding of the structure and politics of memory and transmission, illuminating not just what stories are told, or what images are seen, but how those stories are told and how those images are constructed (Hirsch, *Phototextualities* 23). A feminist analysis allows the critic to consider troubled and troubling narratives of maternal and child conflict, which explore resentment and rejection, as well as familiar sentimental versions of maternal relations. Moreover, the continuing use of the figure of the vulnerable child in the discourse of Indigenous child protection in Australia today, which I discuss in the final section, makes a gendered analysis crucially important.

While Kahane's article raises important issues about the gendering of cultural memories of trauma, there are certain assumptions that need to be addressed to make it relevant to Stolen Generations discourse. Like many trauma critics, Kahane privileges literary discourse as the cultural form most capable of conveying the affect of trauma. She contends that 'through its semiotic strategies of encoding and conveying affect' literary discourse 'can make real and present the inaccessible historical past and the experience of the other' and 'can transmit the texture of traumatic memory' (163-64). In Indigenous Australian culture, memory is typically passed on through vernacular languages such as oral storytelling rather than through literary discourse (Bennett and Kennedy 11). Many narratives of Indigenous child removal have been transcribed from oral interviews and testimonies produced in a collaboration between Indigenous witnesses and Indigenous and non-Indigenous historians, lawyers, and ethnographers. Figurative devices are inevitably used to shape these narratives, but they are usually not 'worked through' to the degree that much Holocaust testimony is (Felman and Laub 5). As Bella Brodzki points out, even within literary discourse, various strategies are used to convey trauma. In some trauma texts the author '... renders an experience of terror, horror, or shame explicitly, directly, almost didactically, perhaps using the word *trauma* itself ... .' (128). In other texts, traumatic memory may be registered linguistically through the structure of the text, and through devices such as figures, flashbacks and repetitions (130). The particular forms that are used to transmit memories of trauma are diverse and shaped by a range of factors, including cultural and linguistic traditions, and generic conventions. In recognition of this cultural diversity, it is important to challenge the widespread claim that literary discourse is uniquely suited to transmit the affect and experience of trauma from victim to secondary witness. It is also worth questioning the assumption that it is possible or desirable to transmit the experience of trauma and loss to others, especially where there are vast differences of culture and experience involved. Perhaps some traumatic experiences can only be acknowledged and survived.

Rabbit-Proof Fence

Philip Noyce's 2002 film *Rabbit-Proof Fence,* an adaptation of Pilkington's narrative, is one of the few Stolen Generations narratives to circulate internationally. A rare escape story, the film follows Molly, Gracie and Daisy as they escape from Moore River Native Settlement, and walk an arduous 1600 kilometres through bush and desert, guided by the rabbit-proof fence, back to home and mother. Together Pilkington's narrative and Noyce's film offer the opportunity to examine how the cultural memory of the Stolen Generations has been mediated, not only by literary and cinematic conventions, but by transnational discourses of trauma and the Holocaust. Not only is the film mediated by the *Bringing Them Home* report (Collins and Davis 133). It aimed to be the *Schindler's List* of the Stolen Generations: a representative story standing for a multitude of other stories. Hughes D'aeth has convincingly argued that *Rabbit-Proof Fence* is 'visually' and 'conceptually linked' to *Schindler's List,* although he does not consider the gendered dimensions of the transnational Holocaust iconography Noyce cites.[13] One of the most striking features of Noyce's adaptation is his use of the maternal trope to construct a powerful cultural memory of the Stolen Generations, and to mediate this story for international audiences. To draw out the contrast between text and film versions, I first consider Pilkington's text.

As someone who was herself forcibly assimilated into white Australian culture as a child, Pilkington occupies a hybrid position, as an insider and outsider to an Aboriginal culture that was irreversibly transformed by colonisation. Reconstructing the story of her mother and aunt's journey from their oral testimonies, archival sources, and her own childhood memories of the landscape surrounding Moore River, she articulates the challenges of translating Aboriginal forms of knowledge for Western readers, while still conveying their cultural specificity and difference (Pilkington 1996, xii). Although she places the story of the girls' removal in the broader context of dispossession and colonisation, she writes in a voice that strives not to accuse. The story opens with a collective mythic Indigenous memory of the arrival of Europeans in the 1800s, and the first settlement in what is now Western Australia. Over time, as a result of dispossession and scarcity of traditional food sources, some Aboriginal clans move into Jigalong, a government depot that offered food and security. Molly and her cousins, the first children of mixed-descent in the area, were taunted by the 'full-blood' children, which was noticed by the depot manager, and communicated to Neville as a reason for removing them. The narrator reports that '[p]olicies were introduced by the government . . . to provide for the welfare and education needs of these children' (40). This passive construction removes responsibility for assimilation policies from any individual, and apparently accepts that they were formulated with benevolent intentions. It is worth recalling, however, that Pilkington's narrative was published before *Bringing Them Home*, when the history and effects of these policies were not widely known or acknowledged by non-Indigenous Australians.

Without apportioning blame, the narrative represents child removal as a devastating and cataclysmic event that affected the whole Aboriginal clan. In the scene in which Molly, Daisy and Gracie are being taken, Officer Riggs explains to the clan that the girls will be sent to school to be educated:

> The old man nodded to show that he understood what Riggs was saying. The rest of their family just hung their heads . . . Molly and Gracie sat silently on the horse, tears streaming down their cheeks . . . . A high pitched wail broke out. The cries of agonised mothers and the women, and the deep sobs of grandfathers, uncles and cousins filled the air . . . . those remaining in the camp found strong sharp objects and gashed themselves and inflicted wounds to their heads and bodies as an expression of their sorrow (44–45).

Grief and despair are conveyed through universal codes such as sobbing and wailing, and through self-inflected wounds to the head, '. . . a customary [Aboriginal] action of the distressed and the anguished' (131). Through such signifiers, the narrative directly represents the grief and social suffering caused by removal. In this scene, the response to removal is neither individualised nor gendered; the whole group participates, and the men as well as women express distress. When Gracie's mother accuses the child's white father of doing nothing to prevent her removal, he reminds her that Gracie is his daughter too, and that he is powerless to prevent her removal.

Pilkington situates child removal in the context of white settlement and the dispossession of Indigenous people from their lands. Noyce, however, focuses on the maternal melodrama. The film begins with text that explains the policy of child removal in Western Australia in 1931, under Chief Protector of Aborigines, A. O. Neville. In the first spoken words of the film, Molly states in dialect: 'This is a true story . . .' As the scene unfolds, the female kin group – Molly, Daisy, Gracie, their mothers and grandmother – converse in dialect, while tracking a goanna. This scene signals the importance of maternal relations in handing on hunting and other survival skills, and an appreciation for country. Observing the group from up on a ridge, Hungerford, the manager of Jigalong depot, identifies the girls for Constable Riggs, who is preparing to remove them. Sometime later, inside a shed, Riggs watches and waits for the children. While their mothers collect rations, the girls chat idly with a young white man who, like their father, works on the rabbit-proof fence. When they suddenly hear a car, the mothers flee, grabbing the children as they run. The sound of a camel roaring and drums beating heightens the emotional intensity. Trapping the women and girls between the fence and his car, Riggs jumps out and violently wrenches the girls away from their mothers. As he shoves them into the car, he waves a piece of paper, shouting: "It's the law Maude . . . .Nothing you can do". She protests violently that they are *her* children, that Molly is going to marry soon, and they belong in their country. Screaming and wailing, the women beat on the windows and chase the car. As it speeds away, the two mothers lie crumpled in the dirt, while the girls' grandmother pounds her head with a rock. Noyce uses these images of grieving mothers and terrified children, struggling with an overpowering paternal authority, to powerful emotional effect. Close-ups invite audiences to identify with the mothers' grief and the children's fear. At the same time, however, the ending of this scene, in which the women perform their abject status by self-harming and lying in the road like corpses, stages an unpalatable and rarely expressed truth that pushes at the limits of the sentimental framing. This tragic scene acknowledges that the government's assimilation policy renders the mothers disposable, easily replaced by other preferred guardians. The "law" not only legitimates the theft of their children; it robs the women of their cultural and legal status as mothers.

While the overwhelming emotional pull of the removal scene is with the mothers and children, it is worth noting that there are two non-Indigenous witnesses in this scene: the depot manager Hungerford, and the fence worker. Hungerford, who knows the girls are about to be taken, remains distanced and impassive during their capture. By contrast, the young fence worker shifts uncomfortably at the margins of the scene, raising his hand to his mouth in an expression of alarm as he watches the girls being torn from their mothers. In his T-shirt and khakis, he appears powerless in the face of the commanding paternal authority of the uniformed Riggs. Through this sympathetic, yet ambiguous figure, the film fleetingly acknowledges, and invites the viewer to acknowledge, the passive complicity of ordinary Australians in Indigenous child removal. Yet, the rhetorical force of the bystander figure is lessened by the sentimental focus on the struggle between Riggs, the girls and their mothers. In contrast, the young man appears only for an instant. For the most part, the film distances viewers from reflecting critically on the compromised positions of the white characters and instead elicits identification with the purity of maternal grief and childhood innocence.

Rabbit Proof Fence ends with the unexpected revelation of repeated trauma, which heightens the intensity of maternal suffering. After weeks of walking and near-death experiences, the girls approach the outskirts of Jigalong at dusk. Constable Riggs hears commotion from the women's camp, which is preparing for the girls' arrival, and goes to investigate. In a scene that conveys the menace of the Australian bush and the 'otherness' of Indigeneity, Riggs is confronted by Molly's mother and grandmother, threatening him with spears. Spooked by the call of a bird, and the rage of the women, he runs off. As dawn breaks, Molly and Daisy are met by their mother and grandmother. In a scene of joyous reunion, laden with pathos, Molly runs into her grandmother's arms. As they embrace, she repeatedly sobs 'I lost one,' a reference to Gracie's recapture. Molly's grief at her 'loss' of Gracie prefigures her later grief at the loss of her own daughter. The film cuts to Neville in his office, acknowledging that he has no further resources to recapture the girls, but asking the depot officer to keep an eye on them for the future.

The next and penultimate scene, which continues the story after the triumphant return of Molly and Daisy to Jigalong, is electrifying. As the camera pans over the bush, viewers hear Molly speaking in dialect. The translation reads:

> Then we went and hid in the desert. Got married. I had 2 baby girls. Then they took me and my kids back to that place, Moore River. And I walked all the way ... back to Jigalong again, carrying Annabelle...When she was 3, that Mr Neville took her away. I've never seen her again. Gracie is dead now. She never made it back to Jigalong.

This analeptic description of Molly's own experience as a mother is shocking enough, but what is not made explicit is that Molly had to leave four-year-old Doris behind when she carried Annabelle to Jigalong. Much of the debate about the film focuses on its sentimentality, which is anchored in maternal tropes, but critics have tended to overlook the film's acknowledgment of the limits of translating trauma across cultural difference.[14] The devastating revelation of repeated trauma is mediated through an Indigenous voice, which is a tribute to Pilkington, who strived to respect Aboriginal knowledge and customs while translating them for non-Indigenous audiences. The linguistic dissonance of the Aboriginal voice—so unexpected in a commercial 'Hollywood' film—signifies the untranslatability of traumatic memory. Molly's voice powerfully conveys the extent to which the affective legacy of trauma cannot be shared, but rather isolates the women. What Holocaust survivor Charlotte Delbo calls the 'sensory memory' of trauma—in this case, perhaps Molly's bodily memory of carrying a toddler 1600km, while grieving for the child she has left behind—is registered, but not 'translated', through Molly's embodied voice.

In the final frames of the film, the real Molly and Daisy, now old women, stand on a hill in Jigalong. Molly says: 'Daisy and me, we're living here in our country. We're never going back to that place' which refers to Moore River, but could also refer to the 'place' of traumatic memory.[15] Structurally, the documentary ending is similar to that of *Schindler's List*, in that both films introduce the real historical figures to reiterate the 'truth' of the narrative, and to bring the legacy of the past into the present. But the affect of the scenes is entirely different. In *Schindler's List*, the survivors, surrounded by their families, confirm their survival and procreation. In *Rabbit-Proof Fence*, the women stand alone, which reminds viewers of those who have not come home. The intense sense of maternal loss, conveyed through Molly's narrative of her stolen daughters and the loss of Gracie, is alleviated only through her connection with the land, which enables survival in the face of the government's relentless assault on Indigenous family bonds. Although the diegetic ending provides closure, with the girls successfully arriving home, the film concludes, through the extra-diegetic ending, without resolution or reconciliation. While *Rabbit Proof Fence* tells only one story, a rare story, it is often curiously taken as representative. Thus, its particular representation of the girls' longing for home and mother is made to stand for a cultural rather than a personal memory of the Stolen Generations, in which nostalgia for home and maternal loss are dominant tropes.

Trauma Narrative from National to Transnational

Use of the maternal trope is further evidenced in the international marketing campaign for the film, which involved the re-packaging of Pilkington's memoir as a tie-in with the film. A reading of the covers of *Rabbit Proof Fence*, from its first edition in 1996 to its most recent edition in 2005, reveals the prevalence of gendered imagery in mediating the shift from a local to a global market, and in constructing a cultural memory of Stolen Generations. These covers are an example of what Gerard Genette calls 'peritexts': those texts that wrap, mediate and give meaning to the main text. In contrast to the Australian vernacular aesthetic signified by the benign pastoral scene on the cover of the first Australian edition of Pilkington's memoir, the global marketing of *Rabbit-Proof Fence* used iconography associated with a gendered visual aesthetic of trauma and distant suffering—drawn from the iconography of the Holocaust, and of refugees escaping from peril. The covers of the 2002 edition of the book, and the DVD, carry a film still of Molly carrying a wounded and emaciated Daisy home. Both girls are dressed in the tattered, shapeless dress of a refugee camp; behind them is a barbed-wire fence. The clouds are an ominous orange and brown, connoting smoke. In the context of the Bosnian and Serbian wars of the 1990s, and the Rwandan genocide, this visual framing of the Stolen Generations links it to international atrocities, and positions it for a global market hungry for stories of trauma and distant suffering.

If the marketing for North American and European audiences rhetorically and visually linked the Stolen Generations to the Holocaust and the global refugee crisis, in Japan the historical and political connotations of the film were downplayed in favour of a sentimental framing. A Japanese advertisement promoted the film as 'a universal story about the separation of mother and child'. The advertisement added an element of adventure: 'I just want to see my mum. There are 1500 km to my hometown, where my mum is waiting.' What makes the story 'universal', of course, is its celebration of the bond between mother and child. If the film's reception in Japan is indicative, *Rabbit Proof Fence* was not widely received as a story about the traumas of colonialism, and how the legacy of dispossession and colonialism continues to impact upon Aboriginal Australians in the present.[16] In 2006, Pilkington produced a children's version of her mother's story, titled *Home to Mother*, which like the Japanese ad, mediates the story through the maternal bond. This commodification and the various iterations of the *Rabbit Proof Fence* narrative, and the iconic status of this particular version of Stolen Generations trauma, disavows the less culturally palatable effects of child removal and assimilation – the ambivalences and potentially irreparable estrangement of the mother-child relation. These are the taboos that Kofman engages with so bravely. So, too, has Doris Pilkington, although her narrative of the estrangement of mother-child bonds that occurred in her own family is less well known.

Unsettling the Maternal Trope

When she died in 2004, Molly said she had 'one regret'—that she did not see her daughter Annabelle again (Collins and Davis 144). In their reading of *Rabbit Proof Fence*, Felicity Collins and Theresa Davis regard Molly's statement as revealing what is 'unspeakable' or 'unrecoverable' in her story– that is, the traumatic loss of her daughter (145). There is, however, another dimension to Molly's story, not available to global or national audiences, that reveals a further layer of trauma that cannot be integrated into a sentimental framing. At a public screening of *Rabbit Proof Fence* in 2005, Pilkington told the audience that she had contacted her sister before their mother died, and told her of their mother's wish to see her. But her sister, for private reasons of her own, did not want to meet her mother or kin, and refused to travel to Jigalong.[17] Her sister's children, who did not know they had Aboriginal family, wanted to meet their relatives. Their mother sent them, with a tin of biscuits, to see their grandmother in Jigalong, who allegedly responded: 'your mother should have brought these herself'. In the ending of the film, Annabelle is figured as a 'lost' child, but in Pilkington's oral commentary she emerges as a 'resistant' adult daughter who refuses to return 'home'. In an unexpected echo of Kofman's memoir, we discover that Molly is not only a bereaved mother but a rejected mother. This anecdotal fragment suggests complexities of experience, emotion and memory that go beyond what can be conveyed through images of suffering mothers and vulnerable children. Pilkington's poignant revelation shocked the audience, confronting us with a concrete case in which the intended aim of the assimilation policy – to pervert and estrange intimate Indigenous family bonds by severing relations between children and their Aboriginal kin – was realized. Her oral commentary reveals the traumatic, intergenerational legacy of child removal: for her mother, unrequited love and life-long suffering; for the daughter and her children, loss of culture and family. This knowledge intensifies the sense of loss associated with the non-redemptive ending of *Rabbit-Proof Fence*, leaving us to ponder the enormous social and personal costs of Indigenous child removal.

In a context in which healing is largely conceptualised as being reunited with lost family, stories about estranged family relations can be impossible to tell. In the current political climate, in which Stolen Generations narratives 'focus on the traumatic effects of forced removals', positive memoirs of removal and assimilation have been greeted with scepticism and charges of denial (Whitlock

31). In this context, the 'lost' daughter's story of why she chose not to return to 'home' and mother may not be welcome. [18] Moreover, the polarised discursive context—in which child removal is interpreted through politicised dichotomies of 'loss' or 'benefit', 'theft' or 'rescue'—makes it difficult to tell stories in which these categories are blurred. The story of the Stolen Generations, as mediated through the maternal trope, is a trauma narrative with which audiences can readily identify.[19] For a non-sentimental rendering of maternal–child relations, it is useful to turn to Kofman's text. How do other dimensions of mother-child relations emerge within Holocaust testimony? What tropes and figures does Kofman use in narrating a story of mother-daughter relations estranged by traumatic events, of the impossibility of returning 'home', and of the difficulties of distinguishing rescue from theft, and protection from abuse?

'The Strange and Estranging Legacy of Trauma': *Rue Ordener, Rue Labat*

Kofman's memoir is grounded in her personal, embodied memory of events, but also informed by her practice as a philosopher who has published on the unspeakability of the Holocaust.[20] As a scholar of Freud's work and an analysand over many years, she writes from within a European tradition of psychoanalysis. She begins *Rue Ordener/Rue Labat* by acknowledging her delay in writing about 'that'—a term which confers the 'unspeakability' of trauma on the memory of her father's deportation and death, and the irrevocable end of family life as she had known it. Yet, she goes on to write about the horror and loss, the betrayal and shame, which cannot be spoken. The text does not linguistically 'act out' traumatic memory through flashbacks and memory fragments; nor is the reader presented with 'bits and pieces of memory overwhelmed by events' (Felman and Laub). Rather, Kofman's style, like that of Primo Levi and Ruth Kluger, is striking for its precision and almost clinical clarity. This clarity suggests a traumatic memory that has been 'radically rethought and fundamentally worked over by the text' (Felman and Laub xiv-xv). The title, which refers to the Parisian streets on which her family and Meme lived, signifies a splitting of the site of 'home' and identity. The memoir succeeds in transmitting the 'strange and estranging legacy of trauma' by revealing how the deportation of her father, the splitting of the family, and her mother's powerlessness in hiding, resulted in a traumatic breach in mother-child relations (Brodzki 129).

The core of Kofman's memoir details the domestic drama played out in hiding. She conveys the intensity of the mother-child bond through repeated scenes in which Sarah acts out her terror of what, as a child, she perceived to be 'the real danger: separation from my mother' (33). She depicts herself, even before her father's arrest, as a highly-strung and often ill child, who suffered from a terror of being abandoned, and who developed strong attachments to mother figures. When her mother hides the children in the country, she refuses to eat pork, and frequently vomits, thereby endangering herself and her siblings.[21] After the roundups intensify, her mother hides her in Paris, with a family, in a hospital, in a boarding house, but she always refused to eat pork, and sobs violently when her mother leaves her. Finally, after nearly leaving her at a monastery which was later raided, her mother decides to keep Sarah with her, until, in February, 1943 'it' happened: they are warned they are 'on the list' for that night. They seek refuge with Meme, who had once been their neighbour (31). The next day Sarah returns with her mother to their flat to find that it has been vandalised by the Gestapo. If, in later life, Kofman feels any nostalgia for her childhood home, it is not conveyed. Rather, her admission—' [n]ever again, except in dreams, have I ever gone back there'—suggests the utter impossibility of a return home, and the profound rupture the Holocaust brought about in Jewish family life (33).

With analytical insight, Kofman describes how a situation of rescue became, for her mother, one of psychological and emotional abuse. Once Sarah and her mother move into Meme's apartment, Sarah's transformation into a 'Christian girl' is set in train. Meme calls her by the Christian name 'Suzanne'. Rather than use food simply to nurture Sarah, Meme uses it as a weapon in her battle against the 'other' mother. Insisting that 'the food of my childhood was unhealthy; I was pale, "lymphatic," I must change my diet' Meme took over caring for Sarah (40). Meme makes her new clothes, supplies her with books, lavishes her with affection, and takes her for walks during which Sarah passes as her daughter. Meme is associated with sensual and illicit bodily pleasures: she kisses Sarah, walks around her apartment bare-chested, and has her lover to spend the night once a week. The young Sarah describes her own reaction to Meme as a kind of seduction: she blushes when she watches Meme undress behind a screen, and welcomes the affection Meme, unlike her own mother, lavishes on her. Kofman recalls how Meme's 'care' led to amnesia:

> I had, it seemed, buried the entire past: I started loving rare steak cooked in butter and parsley. I didn't think any more at all about my father, and I couldn't pronounce a single word of Yiddish despite the fact that I could still understand the language of my childhood perfectly (57).

Kofman does not represent herself as resistant or innocent, but rather as complicit. She recalls how easy she made it for Meme to win her over, and the pain she half-knowingly inflicted on her mother. For instance, she recalls a Mother's Day when, after agonising, she decided to give the more beautiful of the two cards she has bought to Meme. Her wording—'my choice has undeniably been made' (45)—positions her childhood self as aware of her betrayal. Her intense bond with Meme culminates in an episode in which the two go to the country one Sunday to visit Meme's family, and miss the last metro home. They stay in a hotel, and Sarah, who shares a bed with Meme, is 'relieved' not to have to walk the formidable distance to Rue Labat. But her mother looms like a disturbing presence that keeps Sarah from guiltlessly enjoying her pleasure with Meme, as she worried '... about separation from my mother' whom she knows will be frantic (55). Kofman recalls that by the time Paris is liberated, and they come out of hiding, '[m]y mother felt nothing any more but hate and contempt for the woman who'd saved our lives' (58). The feelings of anxiety and dread that Sarah had previously experienced at being separated from her mother are transferred to Meme: 'It tore me in two. Overnight I had to take leave of the woman I now loved more than my own mother' (58). From her child's point of view, she is not liberated but rather subjected to another 'traumatic separation', and consigned to a miserable life in a dirty, crowded hotel with her mother and siblings.

Whereas Kofman remembers her father only lovingly, she recalls incriminating details about her mother (as if she has taken on the role of 'prosecuting' her mother). After they leave Meme's, her mother allows her one-hour visits to ease the transition: 'If I stayed away a second too long, she would beat me with a strap ... I was soon covered with bruises and began to detest my mother ... strangely enough, she had thought to bring that strap with her the day we escaped ...' (59). Her mother sues Meme for having 'tried to "take advantage" of me and of having mistreated [her] ...' (59). In a disturbing inversion of Foigel's testimony, Kofman confesses that she testified against her 'cruel' mother, showing the court her bruises. The court decides to leave Sarah in Meme's care. The guilt she feels manifests itself, as usual, in bodily symptoms (60). When Meme calls her lover Paul to tell him that she won the suit, Sarah's stomach 'was in a knot. I peered around me in the street as if I had just committed a crime—as if once again I were "wanted"' (61). In her recollection of this incident, her mother has become a perpetrator who, like the Nazis, hunts the child down in an effort to steal her from the 'mother' she now loves more than her own. The young Sarah plays the role of the hunted, frequently running away to Meme, flouting her mother's rules and wishes. Yet, she also recalls her ambivalent relief when her mother, accompanied by two burly men, 'steals' her back from Meme. In conveying this episode, in which no one behaves selflessly, Kofman's memoir reveals how the assimilation of the child can lead to the perversion of mother-child relations. Her 'troubling confession' challenges our notions of maternal self-sacrifice and childhood innocence (Brooks). It acknowledges how traumatic experience produces estrangement and alienation in the intimate relations that are, as we have seen, conventionally represented in the most sentimental ways in popular versions of Stolen Generations story.

Kofman mediates her memory of childhood trauma through two cultural narratives of mother-child relations, thereby suggesting this maternal dimension of her memoir might be placed in a broader comparative context. Both these narratives reflect on the mutability of subject positions in contexts of unequal power in intimate relations. The first is a Leonardo da Vinci painting, *Madonna and Child with St. Anne*, in which two women look lovingly at the infant, while an older woman is in the background. When da Vinci's father re-married, his mother was 'replaced' in his affections by his loving step-mother. Freud comments that: "The artist seems to have used the blissful smile of St. Anne to disavow and to cloak the envy which the unfortunate woman felt when she was forced to give up her son to her better-born rival, as she had once given up his father as well" (64). Kofman's memoir of her survival in hiding can also be read as a theft masked through affection and care. Meme uses the pretext of offering 'protection' to disavow her anti-Semitism; she masks her cruel behaviour to Sarah's mother's by offering to 'ease' her burden.

The second example is Kofman's discussion of a scene from Alfred Hitchcock's film, *The Lady Vanishes*, in which the good little old lady, Mrs. Froy, is replaced by another woman pretending to be her. Kofman says her 'agony is excruciating' when the young woman who had been talking to Mrs Froy, and who has been knocked unconscious, is half-convinced by a pseudo-doctor that she only imagined Mrs. Froy was there, and the other woman had always been there. Kofman interprets this scene as a story about good and bad mothers and the difficulty of telling the two apart: 'The bad breast in place of the good, the one utterly separate from the other, the one changing into the other' (66). Whereas in the Da Vinci painting the child is unaware of events, in this scene the young woman, here representing Kofman's own position, is suspicious that she has been duped—that the good Mrs. Froy has been replaced by an evil woman. Using this scene to mediate her memory of her 'improper' childhood feelings towards her 'two mothers', Kofman suggests the impossibility of making easy or clear distinctions between 'good' and 'bad' mothers, and between 'beneficiaries' and 'victims'. Her mother is not only the suffering mother, but also the cruel mother. Meme is not simply a saviour; she is also an opportunist and beneficiary. Sarah is not simply the innocent child, but the accusing and complicit child; not simply the 'stolen' child but the child who gains pleasure from a new intimate relationship. Rather than provide closure, Kofman ends her memoir with the unapologetic confession that she did not attend Meme's funeral—another acknowledgment of the estranging legacy of trauma. Anti-heroic and unsentimental, her memoir makes uncomfortable reading as there is no apparent reconciliation, no atonement, no forgiveness, only bitterness, regret and guilt.

The debate on the 'limits of representation' often turns on what can be visually represented in Holocaust cinema. Kofman's memoir draws attention to other unspoken limits of representation—particularly regarding mother-child relations. Unlike *Rabbit-Proof Fence*, which invites identification with the mothers and children, Kofman's memoir distances the readers, and calls for critical reflection rather than empathy and identification. With whom would the reader wish to identify in this memoir about the seductions of assimilation, cruel mothers, a defiant daughter, and the difficulties of reparation? Like Ruth Kluger's memoir, *Still Alive: A Holocaust Girlhood Remembered*, Kofman's memoir contributes to a literary tradition of intimate trauma memoir in which mothers and daughters do not behave heroically or selflessly. These unforgiving memoirs, in which memory surfaces through bile, confront the reader with psychological legacies and moral shortcomings that we deal with in denial. These complex and painful realities have not been integrated into the cultural memory of the Stolen Generations, but as we have seen, circulate in the margins – such as in Pilkington's oral commentary.

Conclusion: Legacies of Post/Colonial Trauma in the 21st Century

Rabbit Proof Fence represents Indigenous child removal as a past event. As recent events suggest, however, the traumatic legacy of child removal, dispossession and colonisation continues to be acted out in Indigenous communities. Ten years after *Bringing Them Home*, the discourses and subject positions the assimilation policy produced – particularly that of the vulnerable child and its counterpart, the state as stern but benevolent father – have achieved new potency. In June 2007, the Northern Territory government issued a report, *Little Children Are Sacred*, which documented shocking cases of child sexual abuse in remote Indigenous communities. As the report's title indicates, the figure of the vulnerable child is a recurrent and emotive signifier in the discourse of child protection. In response to the report, the federal government, led by then Prime Minister John Howard, declared a state of 'national emergency'. Howard and his Indigenous Affairs Minister Mal Brough devised a controversial plan of action that became known as the 'Northern Territory Intervention'. Taking what could be described as a 'muscular humanitarian' approach, the government spent millions, bringing in the army, police, bureaucrats and teams of medical personnel to conduct child health checks and curb lawlessness.[22]

From its inception, the intervention divided the Indigenous community and its supporters.[23] While Social Justice Commissioner Tom Calma saw the intervention as an assault on Indigenous rights, Aboriginal leader Noel Pearson used the trope of the 'terrified child huddled in the corner' to garner support for the intervention.[24] Much has changed since the intervention began: Howard lost power in November 2007, and Kevin Rudd, who became prime minister, offered a long-awaited national apology to members of the Stolen Generations in February 2008. The extensive media, academic and policy commentary and analysis of the intervention has revealed that the scope and depth of problems in remote Indigenous communities[0] – alcohol and drug abuse, lawlessness, suicide, poor health, education and child neglect, lack of job opportunities – go far beyond child sexual abuse, and defy easy solutions. The Rudd government, which supported the intervention, is currently undertaking a review to determine its future. Although I cannot discuss the discourses surrounding the intervention in depth, I will tie together the threads of my argument by considering some of the effects of the trope of the vulnerable child, and the legacy of post/colonial trauma in the 21st century.

One of the first newspaper articles to report the intervention used a striking image – a paternal inversion of the maternal trope – to mediate the story (Coorey et al).[25] This image is significant because it anticipated the main fault line in the debate about the intervention: paternalistic opportunism or legitimate 'practical' solution to a dire situation? Covering the top half of a page in the *Sydney Morning Herald*, the image consisted of a windblown Aboriginal flag, frayed at the edges. Inside the yellow circle of the flag is a cropped photograph of then Prime Minister Howard, wearing an Akubra, holding an Aboriginal female toddler.[26] Howard, representative of the authority and power of the state, is positioned as the 'father' of the nation and protector of Aboriginal children. Mediated by the Aboriginal flag, and cropped to focus on the father/child dyad, the photograph invites readers to link the intervention with the Stolen Generations, thereby framing the government's strategy as paternalistic and denying Aboriginal rights. On another reading, the frayed flag suggests that Indigenous communities are in need of urgent help, with the state positioned as legitimate protector of the children. What is telling, for the argument I have been developing, is the replacement of the Indigenous mother (as featured on the cover of *Bringing Them Home*) by the white 'father', once again positioning her as dispensable. In discursive terms, the Indigenous mother is locked into an oppositional binary with the Indigenous male, who has been positioned, in the intervention discourse, as a sexual predator.[27] Thus, Indigenous women are positioned as either 'protecting' the men (rather than the children), and thus opposed to the intervention, or in need of protection from Indigenous male violence, and thus as supporting the intervention. In either case, the threat to indigenous children has been figured as coming primarily from within Indigenous communities – a major shift in the discourse from the National Inquiry, which documented extensive child abuse by non-Indigenous caretakers.[28]

As the above image indicates, the discourse of the intervention has focused almost exclusively on the needs of the 'vulnerable child', considering other members of the community primarily in relation to the child. For instance, in the newspaper article accompanying the image, Howard's rhetorical use of 'little children' lends moral support to the intervention: "I am distressed ... Little children. It is a disgrace that a section of the Australian population, that little children should be the subject of serious sexual abuse" (Coorey et al). As the Northern Territory report makes clear, however, it is not only little children who are suffering and at risk; adults are suffering too, and desperately need help: 'The inquiry found a deeply entrenched and self-sustaining cycle of abuse and violence which had become an inheritance, passing from one generation to the next' (Coorey et al). Illustrating the repetitive nature of trauma, the article quotes testimony by a jailed rapist: "When I was six my old man shot my mum ... bang in the head. They had been blueing all night. He made me clean her brains off the floor. When I raped that girl I felt like all my pain was going into her, when she screamed, that was me screaming" (Coorey et al). This horrific testimony documents an intergenerational cycle of trauma, which is too rarely acknowledged – in part because it is seen as providing excuses for perpetrators. The belief that acknowledging causes of violence, including historical causes, is to excuse violence operates as a firm limit in the intervention discourse, which blocks recognition of the repetitive cycle of trauma.

Like Sarah Kofman in her memoir, Indigenous professor Judy Atkinson, who works on trauma and healing in Indigenous communities, recognises the difficulty of making clear-cut distinctions between 'victim', 'perpetrator', 'collaborator' and 'beneficiary'. With an awareness of the rhetorical power of the figure of the child, Atkinson positions the 'rapist' as someone who was once a vulnerable child. Identifying a major problem that limits long-term healing, she asks: "How many skilled people do we have in Australia who can work with *that child*, to intervene to stop *that child* raping when he grows up? There aren't many" (Coorey et al, my italics). Whereas Howard focused on the 'little child' in isolation from other members of the community, Atkinson's point is that 'perpetrators' must be treated, not simply excluded or penalised, if the cycle of violence is to be reduced. Speaking of the rapist, she comments: "When a child is that deeply traumatised, he becomes rewired, he can't study ... We need to put healing into the curriculum" (Coorey et al 25). Mick Dodson also points to the need for treatment: "The prohibition of alcohol —that doesn't work because we have to deal with ... the addiction. We've got to give these people support, counselling" (Coorey et al 25).[29] These Indigenous leaders are not opposed to the intervention. They recognise, however, that traumatic events have a tendency to repeat, and produce legacies that cannot be resolved only through practical solutions such as monitoring welfare payments and school attendance, although such policies are part of a solution. Post-trauma counselling is also part of a practical solution, but it requires massive resources which are scarce. Pilkington's oral commentary and Kofman's memoir are important in the context of the national emergency, in that they make us aware of the estranging and repetitive legacy of trauma. If more lives are not to be wasted, implicitly regarded as disposable, a response must recognise the intergenerational repetition of trauma, and provide resources for treatment and healing to all members of the community.

Notes

[1] For discussions of Kofman's memoir in relation to her philosophy, see Deutscher and Oliver; Oliver; and Chanter.

[2] Suicides often prompt a re-reading of an author's earlier works in light of this final act; on Kofman's suicide, see (Robson 616-617), (Deutsche and Oliver 8) and (Dobie vii-xiv).

[3] The late psychoanalyst Dori Laub has argued that, to stop acting out a traumatic event, the survivor needs to integrate the memory fragments into a narrative, which will aid survival. He maintains that the therapeutic process of the 're-externalization of the event can occur and take effect only when one can articulate and transmit the story, literally transfer it to another outside oneself and then take it back again, inside' (Felman and Laub 69). He proposes that Holocaust survivors 'needed to tell their story in order to survive' (Felman and Laub 78).

[4] My account is indebted to Golasan.

[5] The claim that 'stolen generations' testimonies penetrated the heart of non-Indigenous Australia in the way other Indigenous issues had not is frequently repeated. At the tenth anniversary of *Bringing Them Home* at Parliament House, Canberra, on May 27, 2007, an Indigenous speaker commented that unlike other Aboriginal issues, the 'stolen generations' had generated intense empathy among non-Indigenous Australians 'because everyone has a mother ... and everyone has been a child.' Author's personal observation.

[6] I have explored some of the diverse ways in which non-Indigenous Australians have responded to stolen generations testimony in Kennedy 2004.

[7] See the essays in Curthoys and Docker, and Moses.

[8] I may be regarded as doing violence to Kofman's text by reading it in a context so foreign to her own interests, but I believe this is one of the possibilities generated by a transnational Holocaust memory discourse – that is enables comparisons that may not seem 'appropriate' but that may produce new insights.

[9] Since I am primarily concerned with reading Kofman's memoir in an Australian context, where the English translation is more readily available than the French original, I have quoted from the English.

[10] Barbara Creed reads *Jedda* retrospectively as a 'stolen child' narrative, which presents for viewers today the uncomfortable issue of whether the white 'adopting' mother had any right to remove baby Jedda from her people and raise her as a 'white' child.

[11] For a powerful analysis of the position of the beneficiary in the South African Truth and Reconciliation Commission, see Schaffer and Smith.

[12] Pilkington (2002) has also published a memoir of her childhood and early adulthood, her unlearning of internalised racism, and her journey to Jigalong to find her family.

[13] As D'aeth observers:

> Both films are based on non-fictional accounts ... of traumatic events that were founded on survivor testimony ... they are both survival stories that take place against a backdrop of non-survival ... escape stories that confound a more general condition of imprisonment. Each film also seems conditioned by the expectation that they are bringing their respective traumatic events to "the world" and present themselves implicitly as representative of a multitude of similar stories.

[14] For a range of views on the film's sentimentality, see Birch; Potter and Schaffer; and D'aeth. Collins and Davis argue that the ending of the film positions spectators as witnesses to Indigenous trauma.

[15] This scene recalls a scene in Claude Lanzmann's film, *Shoah*, in which one of the witnesses, Mordecai Polchebank, when asked what he feels about the horrors he witnessed in the Holocaust, responds: "I don't go back there".

[16] In marketing the film exclusively through the maternal trope, an opportunity was missed to draw attention to the struggle of Japan's indigenous peoples, the Ainu, who like Australian Aborigines have suffered from oppression, dispossession and child removal.

[17] Screening and discussion of *Rabbit-Proof Fence* with Doris Pilkington, National Library of Australia, 2005. Author's personal observation.

[18] Jay Arthur, a curator the National Museum of Australia, has discussed with me the difficulties of telling complex stories of removal, which might be seen to challenge the dominant narrative of traumatic separation (Kennedy 2008). See also Schaffer; Hosking.

[19] LaCapra argues that an empathic response to victims should not foreclose or become a substitute for 'attempts to work through the past and its losses, both in victims ... and in secondary witnesses' (47). See also his discussion on pp. 212–213.

[20] Kofman first wrote about the Holocaust and her father's deportation and death in *Smothered Words*, published in French in 1987. After this text, as Dobie notes, Judaism, anti-Semitism, the Shoah, and autobiography emerged as 'predominant concerns' in her work. Dobie describes Kofman's anti-sentimental approach: "by presenting the events [of her father's deportation] as a set of statistics, she banished the potential for pathos and avoids any attempt to describe or explain. She also underscores the fact that what she is describing is an historical as well as a personal trauma" (xi-xii).

[21] Robson offers a compelling analysis of the figure of the vomiting body in Kofman's memoir.

[22] On muscular humanitarism, see Orford. The health checks were originally intended as 'forensic exams' to determine the extent of child sex abuse. In response to an outcry, including by doctors, the health checks were made voluntary, and did not seek evidence of sexual abuse. See *Lateline* interview with Mal Brough, aired on 20/6/2008, available at: http://www.abc.net.au/lateline/content/2007/s2281522.htm

[23] For some of the extensive ABC coverage of the Northern Territory Intervention, see '*Lateline*' and '*Breakfast*' archives on http://www.abc.net.au , and see *Four Corners*, 'Tracking the Intervention', broadcast on 5/11/2007, available at http://www.abc.net.au/4corners/content/2007/s2079819.htm For analysis of and critical responses to the National Emergency, see Altman and Hinkson, and Langton.

[24] Pearson used the emotive figure of 'the child huddled in the corner' in an interview with Fran Kelley on Radio National *Breakfast*, 20 June 2007, at http://www.abc.net.au/rn/breakfast/stories/2007/1956365.htm - 6k - [html] - 20 Jun 2007. Tom Calma responded on the same show the following day: www.abc.net.au/rn/breakfast/stories/2007/1956365.htm - 6k - [html] - 21 Jun 2007. The figure of the vulnerable child has been taken up by conservative commentators such as *The Australian* columnist Janet Albrechtson to defend the government intervention plan against charges of 'paternalism' and 'racial discrimination'.

[25] I would like to thank Sue Andrews for drawing this article to my attention.

[26] Three months later, in an article discussing Howard's shock announcement that, if re-elected, he would hold a referendum to recognise Indigenous Australians in a preamble to the Constitution, *The Australian* printed the photograph from which the figure of Howard holding the child was cropped. In the photograph, taken in 2005, Howard is visiting a Northern Territory community, and is surrounded by children of all ages.

[27] At the October 13, 2007 opening of the 'Culture Warriors' Indigenous art exhibit at the National Gallery of Australia, artist Vernon Ah Kee wore a black T-shirt which read: "I do not bash women": In his talk, he objected to the government's discourse on Northern Territory communities, which positioned all Indigenous men as rapists, paedophiles, alcoholics and wife-beaters. Author's personal observation.

[28] In the article accompanying the image, the journalist comments that Judy Atkinson "knows the self-perpetuating nature of the problem [of sexual abuse]. She herself, a Jiman woman from Central Queensland, was sexually abused as a child by a [white?] church official". This important detail reminds readers that perpetrators use positions of authority to gain access to children, and come from outside as well as within Indigenous communities.

[29] In an essay on Indigenous male violence, Greer (2008) argues that it is important to treat the 'underlying pathology'. Also see her interview with Fran Kelly on Radio National *Breakfast*, August 14, 2008: http://www.abc.net.au/rn/breakfast/stories/2008/2334875.htm

References

Altman, Jon and Melinda Hinkson, eds. *Coercive Reconciliation: Stabilise, Normalise, Exit Aboriginal Australia*. Melbourne: Arena Publications, 2007.

Anderson, Patricia and Rex Wild, QC. *Little Children Are Sacred: Report of the Northern Territory Board of Inquiry into the Protection of Aboriginal Children from Sexual Abuse* (2007).

Bennett, Jill and Rosanne Kennedy. 'Introduction.' *World Memory: Personal Trajectories in Global Time*. Ed. Jill Bennett and Rosanne Kennedy. London: Palgrave-Macmillan, 2003.

Birch, Tony. 'This is a True Story: *Rabbi-Proof Fence*, 'Mr Devil' and the Desire to Forget'. *Cultural Studies Review*. 8.1 (2002): 117–129.

Brodzki, Bella. 'Trauma and Transmission.' *Teaching the Representation of the Holocaust*. Ed. Marianne Hirsch and Irene Kacandes. New York, N.Y: Modern Language Association of America, 2004.

Brooks, Peter. *Troubling Confessions: Speaking Guilt in Law and Literature*. Chicago: University of Chicago Press, 2000.

Collins, Felicity, and Theresa, Davis. *Australian Cinema After Mabo*. Cambridge, U.K.; New York: Cambridge University Press, 2004.

Chanter, Tina. 'Eating Words: Antigone as Kofman's Proper Name'. *Enigmas: Essays on Sarah Kofman*. Ed. Penelope Deutscher and Kelly Oliver. New York: Cornell University Press, 1999.

Coorey, Phillip, Peter Hartcher and Stephanie Peatling. 'Just Imagine if it was Marrickville: Why the Prime Minister Took Control'. *The Sydney Morning Herald: Weekend Edition*, June 23–25, 2007: 25.

Creed, Barbara. 'Breeding Out the Black: *Jedda* and the Stolen Generations in Australia'. *Body Trade: Captivity, Cannibalism and Colonialism in the Pacific*. Ed. Barbara Creed and Jeanette Hoorn. New York: Routledge, 2001.

Curthoys, Ann and John Docker, eds. Special section on 'Genocide'. *Aboriginal History*. 26 (2001).

D'aeth, Tony Hughes. 'Which Rabbit-Proof Fence? Empathy, Assimilation, Hollywood.' *Australian Humanities Review* (2002). //www.lib.latrobe.edu.au/AHR/archive/Issue-September-2002/hughesdaeth.htm >.

Deutscher, Penelope and Kelly Oliver. 'Introduction: Sarah Kofman's Skirts'. *Enigmas: Essays on Sarah Kofman*. Ed. Penelope Deutscher and Kelly Oliver. New York: Cornell University Press, 1999.

Dobie, Madeleine. 'Translator's Introduction'. *Smothered Words*. Sarah Kofman. Trans. by Madeleine Dobie. Evanston: Northwestern University Press, 1998.

Felman, Shoshana, and Dori Laub. *Testimony: Crises of Witnessing in Literature, Psychoanalysis, and History*. New York and London: Routledge, 1992.

Genette, Gérard. *Paratexts: Thresholds of Interpretation*. Trans. Jane E. Lewis. Cambridge; New York, NY, USA: Cambridge University Press, 1997.

Golasan, Richard J. 'The Legacy of World War II in France: Mapping the Discourses of Memory.' *The Politics of Memory in Postwar Europe*. Ed. Richard Ned Lebow, Wulf Kansteiner, and Claudio Fogu. Durham and London: Duke University Press, 2006.

Greer, Germaine. *On Rage*. Melbourne: Melbourne University Press, 2008.

Hirsch, Marianne. 'Nazi Photographs in Post-Holocaust Art: Gender as an Idiom of Memorialization.' *Phototextualities: Intersections of Photography and Narrative*. Ed. Alex Hughes and Andrea Noble. 2003.

Hosking, Sue. Homeless at Home, Stolen and Saved: Three Colebrook Autobiographies. *Westerly*. 46 (2001): 65–73.

Kahane, Claire. 'Dark Mirrors: A Feminist Reflection on Holocaust Narrative and the Maternal Metaphor.' *Feminist Consequences: Theory for the New Century*. Ed. Elisabeth Bronfen and Misha Kavka. New York: Columbia University Press, 2001.

Kennedy, Rosanne. 'The Affective Work of Stolen Generations Testimony: From the Archives to the Classroom'. *Biography*. 27.1 (2004): 48–77.

———. 'Subversive Witnessing: Mediating Indigenous Testimony in Cultural and Legal Institutions in Australia.' *Women's Studies Quarterly*. 36.1 & 2 (2008): 58–75.

Kluger, Ruth. *Still Alive: a Holocaust Girlhood Remembered*. New York: Feminist Press at the City University of New York, 2001.

Kofman, Sarah. *Rue Ordener, Rue Labat*. Paris: Editions Galilee, 1994.
———. *Rue Ordener, Rue Labat*. Trans. Ann Smock. Lincoln and London: University of Nebraska Press, 1996.
———. *Smothered Words*. Trans. Madeleine Dobie. Evanston: Northwestern University Press, 1998.
LaCapra, Dominick. *Writing History, Writing Trauma*. Baltimore: The Johns Hopkins University Press, 2001.
Levi, Neil. '"No Sensible Comparison"? The Place of the Holocaust in Australia's History Wars'. *History & Memory* 19.1 (2007): 124–156.
Langton, Marcia. 'Trapped in the Aboriginal Reality Show'. *Griffith Review*. 19 (2008).
Link-Up NSW Aboriginal Corporation and Tikka Jan Wilson. *In the Best Interest of the Child?* Canberra, A.C.T.: Aboriginal History, 1997.
Moses, A. Dirk. 'The Holocaust and Genocide.' *The Historiography of the Holocaust*. London: Palgrave Macmillan, 2004.
Noyce, Philip, Dir. *Rabbit-Proof Fence*. Australia, 2002.
Oliver, Kelly. 'Sarah Kofman's Queasy Stomach and the Riddle of the Paternal Law'. *Enigmas: Essays on Sarah Kofman*. Eds. Penelope Deutscher and Kelly Oliver. New York: Cornell University Press, 1999.
Orford, Anne. 'Muscular Humanitarianism: Reading the Narratives of the New Interventionism'. *EJIL*. 10.4 (1999): 679–711.
Pilkington Garimara, Doris. *Follow the Rabbit-Proof Fence*. St. Lucia, Queensland: University of Queensland Press, 1996.
Pilkington Garimara, Doris. *Under the Wintamarra Tree*. St. Lucia, Queensland: University of Queensland Press, 2002.
Pine, Lisa. 'Gender and the Family.' *The Historiography of the Holocaust*. London: Palgrave Macmillan, 2004.
Potter, Emily and Kay Schaffer. '*Rabbit-Proof Fence*, Relational Ecologies and the Commodification of Indigenous Experience.' *Australian Humanities Review*. 31–32 (2004). http://www.lib.latrobe.edu.au/AHR/archive/Issue-April-2004/schaffer.html.
Robson, Kathryn. 'Bodily Detours: Sarah Kofman's Narratives of Childhood Trauma.' *Modern Language Review*. 99.3 (2004): 608–621.
Schaffer, Kay. 'Narrative Lives and Human Rights; Stolen Generation Narratives and the Ethics of Recognition.' *Journal of the Association for the Study of Australian Literature*. 3 (2004): 5–36.
Schaffer, Kay and Sidonie Smith. 'Human Rights, Storytelling, and the Position of the Beneficiary: Antjie Krog's *Country of My Skull*.' *PMLA*. 121.5 (2006): 1577–1584.
Shanahan, Dennis. 'Howard's Open Door'. *Weekend Australian*, October 13–14, 2007: 19–20.
Suleiman, Susan Rubin. 'The 1.5 Generation: Thinking About Child Survivors and the Holocaust.' *American Imago*. 59.3 (2002): 277–295.
Wieviorka, Annette. *The Era of the Witness*. Ithaca, NY: Cornell Univ. Press, 2006.
Whitlock, Gillian. 'Active remembrance: testimony, memoir and the work of reconciliation.' *Rethinking Settler Colonialism: History and Memory in Australia, Canada, Aotearoa New Zealand and South Africa*. Ed. Annie E. Coombes. Manchester and New York: Manchester University Press, 2006.
Wilson, Sir Ronald. Ed. *Bringing Them Home: Report of the National Inquiry into the Separation of Aboriginal and Torres Strait Islander Children from Their Families*. Sydney: Human Rights and Equal Opportunity Commission, 1997.

For comments on previous drafts of this article, I would like to thank Kate Douglas, Gillian Whitlock, Sue Andrews, Jeanette Hoorn and Rosemary Jolly. For inviting me to present this work and generously engaging with it, I would like to thank Mark Phillips, Ruth Phillips, Barbara Gabriel, and their graduate students in Cultural Mediations at Carleton University; the Centre for Research and Teaching on Women at McGill; and the audience at the 'Testimony and Witness' conference at the Australian National University.

Letters from Nauru

Gillian Whitlock

Entering the Epistolarium

In a relatively slender file in the first of the four boxes that archive the Julian Burnside/Kate Durham collection of letters from Nauru, we find a photograph of asylum seeker NRO–2-Y001 yellow.[1] He sent this photograph to Kate Durham early in 2003, and the envelope archived with this photograph gives his address: Top Side camp, Nauru, Central Pacific. He writes on his own account: 'I know a little English and I am sending this letter with my own words ... My name is Bowman Ali my ID is NRO 2 yellow 001 I got letter by your name I am not sure if it was for me but I am replying to you ... It is like I am hanging in the air and nowhere to go, perhaps you could help me make my decision'. His choice is stark: his claim for refugee status has been rejected, he can remain in permanent detention on Nauru, or accept a $2,000 bounty and repatriation to Kabul, Afghanistan. It is symptomatic of Nauru letters that an asylum seeker writes in response to a letter that was perhaps not addressed to him, that we cannot know if these words were written by him or transcribed by an amanuensis in the camp, and he speaks of ongoing and traumatic loss and uncertainty.

The traces of Bowman Ali that remain are this photograph, three letters and two cards and five envelopes in one of forty-eight folders of letters from Nauru which are now in the Burnside/Durham collection recently purchased by the

Fryer library at the University of Queensland. This image is a point of reference to enter this collection, and to find a way around and through the mass of letters exchanged between asylum seekers held on Nauru as part of the Pacific Solution introduced by the Howard government in 2001, and the activists who campaigned on their behalf as part of the 'Spare Rooms for Refugees' project initiated by the artist Durham and her partner the Melbourne QC Julian Burnside. The concept I will use to grapple with this mass of letters is 'the epistolarium'. Liz Stanley introduces this to suggest a rich and varied methodology for mapping collections of letters and their dynamics, including the specific uses of the epislolary form, the voice created by the writers and the space created for the recipient in dialogical exchange, and the specific ethics that emerge within the epistolary community. Stanley's working example of the epistolarium is the archive of Olive Schreiner letters, and obviously the letters from Nauru are a very different example—they emerge from an apocalyptic experience of trauma in a quite precise historical and political context. Nevertheless, Stanley's approach to letters as theatres for the construction and performance of self by the writer and the recipient as a 'mutual metonymy' (212) and intersubjective exchange, sets the stage for the complex cross-cultural relations that are mediated through these letters from Nauru.

These letters find a place in what I have characterised in *Soft Weapons* as a new era for testimony that emerged after 9/11, drawing in part on Derek Gregory's characterisation of 'the colonial present'. The series of interrelated events gathered together as the 'war on terror' produced conditions, routes and discursive formations for the production and transfer of testimony and the emotional and intellectual work of giving witness.[2] Life narrative rapidly became caught up variously in the ideological shifts associated with the war on terror: the renewal of fundamentalisms, the resurgence of homelands and patriotism, the renewed vigor of orientalism and occidentalism in the constructions of self and other, a pervasive strengthening of the modes of state power that operate diffusely to regulate populations and produce docile subjects, and the appropriation of human rights discourse by the state. The war on terror rippled through life narrative with political effect and emotional affect, and it has made work on life narrative and human rights more urgent and difficult than ever before. This is the wider context for these letters. Initiated by the Howard government in September 2001, the Pacific Solution was a state sanctioned policy of brutality, degradation and dehumanisation of asylum seekers driven by the rhetoric of defending the integrity of the sovereign state.

In the wake of all this, we must make more substantial claims for the social, political, cultural and personal significance of life narrative. By characterising life narrative as a 'soft weapon', I want to emphasise its power to humanise categories of people whose experiences are frequently unseen and unheard—to attend to a feminist militant body beneath a burqa, to attach a face and recognise an asylum seeker as an individual with human rights is to make a powerful intervention in debates about social justice, sovereignty and human rights. Life narrative can do these things. But it is also easily co-opted into propaganda—the careful management of information in the engineering of consent. Life narrative is implicated in what will and will not count as viable speaking subjects, the constant creation of what it means to be human and the rights that fall from that, the ongoing negotiation of imaginary boundaries between ourselves and others, and debates about what constitutes a reasonable opinion in the public domain. Testimony above all, mediates the transits of life story across cultures, and the constant creation and recreation of identity and difference in an ongoing and dynamic process. The reality of certain lives and deaths fall from this production, circulation and recognition of testimony, these deliberations about who counts as human, whose lives count as lives and—to use Judith Butler's phrase—what makes for a grievable life. This struggle is at the heart of the Nauru epistolarium: these letters stake a claim to human rights in defiance of a policy that specifically denies asylum seekers a face, a name and a humanising presence. In these circumstances, the letter has unique power and force as a testimonial artifact. As an instrument of cross-cultural exchange that intersubjectivity and mutual metonymy that Stanley remarks upon assumes particular force. This epistolarium draws together a complex series of texts and intertexts, images and artifacts and objects that together give testimony to trauma.

The Careers of the Afghan Girl

The photograph of Bowman Ali presents an intertext quite explicitly and, ironically, it is this figure that draws me to him and shapes a point of entry into the Nauru epistolarium. The photograph shows the asylum seeker sitting in the quarters at Nauru, and placed alongside him is a drawing of an iconic image called 'the Afghan girl'. It is a haunting picture of an unveiled adolescent girl with sea green eyes that was taken at Nasir Bagh refugee camp in Peshawar in 1984. This is the most famous image of a refugee, and it has been reproduced many times in *National Geographic*—most recently in one of the 100 best pictures portfolio in 2006. On its first appearance in 1984, it was framed in *National Geographic* as a condemnation of the Soviet invasion of Afghanistan.[3]

She appeared again on the cover of *National Geographic* in 2002; symptomatically this coincided with the beginning of Operation Enduring Freedom in Afghanistan. The photographer, Steve McCurry returned to the refugee camps in Peshawar to find the Afghan Girl and attach a name and identity to the face. As Susan Sontag suggests, the photographer's intentions do not determine or stabilise the meaning of the photograph, which will have its own career, blown by the whims and loyalties of the diverse communities that have use for it (35). The picture of the Afghan refugee circulates as one of the iconic images that accrues various meanings and symbolic power that far exceeds its ostensible subject. In 2002, the urgency to return and attach a name, to personalise the Afghan girl, coincides with the appearance of Afghan women in those public spectacles of unveiling in the western media that placed extraordinary symbolic significance on the faces of Afghan women. In the context of the war on terror, this image takes on new life; two decades after her first capture, the image of the Afghan girl resurfaces and she is identified as Sharbat Gula, a Pashtun rural woman, a wife and a mother. The photographer McCurry remarks: 'Afghanistan has been in the Dark Ages for two decades. That she's resurfaced now is perhaps prophetic, a hopeful sign.' (n.p.) Now, McCurry and the *National Geographic* team negotiate for another picture. Her face now is haggard, testifying to grief, pain and hardship. This time Sharbat Gula is interviewed, and she says some confronting things: her life under the Taliban was better, and a time of peace and order. She values the burqa as beautiful thing to wear, not a curse.

The Afghan girl image reminds us that moments when an Afghan person is individualised and humanised are always strategic. The question of how and when 'we' become emotionally attached to the bodies of Afghan children, women and men is an important one. When do we recognise life narratives that give face and authority to their lives? Denying the humanity of asylum seekers is a standard protocol in the mass media, denying the human referent of the face and body at all costs is a response to threat: as unwelcome strangers, asylum seekers threaten the integrity of the nation, these people lose face and become ghosts, and objects of fear and disgust. To accrue value and jurisdiction testimony needs fortune, history and national interest on its side. Afghan asylum seekers who moved south to escape the Taliban and the surge of Operation Enduring Freedom in 2001–2002 had none of these things, and in Australia their appeals for human rights were contested by renewed discourses of belonging: homelands, patriots, closed borders and national security. These were framed in the policy called the Pacific Solution. Asylum seekers are subjected to mandatory detention when they arrive in Australia—this is not new—however, the Pacific Solution established offshore centres in other Pacific nations, such as Nauru and Manus Island PNG, where asylum seekers were held and processed by various agencies: DIMIA, the Department of Immigration and Multicultural Affairs for Australia, IOM, the International Organisation for Migration, and UNHCR, the United Nations High Commission for Refugees. These acronyms recur in letters from Nauru, unpacked into the bureaucratic agencies that process the asylum seekers, and into local functionaries—translators, agents and health workers who are sometimes networked into the ethnic and racial prejudices that discriminate against Hazaras in particular.[4] The Pacific Solution policy held over a thousand asylum seekers offshore, stateless and silenced in deterritorialised camps with no access to media or legal services or human rights advocates, and little access to the Internet or computers. Letters were one of the few resources available to them, yet transcribing their experiences into legible English, locating the addresses of recipients and transcribing them onto envelopes, and acquiring stamps required determination and luck. Nauru letters in many cases grasp the traumatic experiences of asylum seekers who never write letters and cannot read them either. The exchange of the letters, photographs and gifts now held in the Burnside Durham archive was a means of agency and resistance for the asylum seekers and the Australian citizens[5] who are shamed by what was being done to preserve the integrity of the nation, ostensibly in their name.[6] These are not dead letters, they remain powerful incarnations of bodies that were dehumanised and rendered abject, and their addressees who gave witness to their trauma and responded in benevolence and shame. In fact, letters are uniquely well placed to grasp the dynamics of this Pacific carceral archipelago of Nauru, Manus and Christmas Islands.[7]

Nauru letters incarnate the social, cultural, material, temporal and spatial reality of Afghan asylum seekers *and* the unstable grounds of this correspondence. This is signalled in that reincarnation of the Afghan girl in Ali Bowman's Nauru letter—further signs of—to return to Sontag—'its own career, blown by the whims and loyalties of the diverse communities that have use for it.' (35) We see the labour of crafting this image here, translating it to a new set of circumstances. We can only speculate about meanings of this image within Afghan communities in detention and in refugee camps, and Bowman Ali's own self-projection here.

The career of this image reveals entangled and varied uses: Sharbat Gula challenges the doxa of Western liberation that shapes her celebrity, yet again in 2002 the appearance of her image produces generous donations for a fund to educate Afghan girls. In 2002 as in 1984, there is the coalescence of state policy and humanitarianism in her name. For Bowman Ali, the drawing might signal his civility in including this artwork in his photograph—it is not incidental after all, but carefully placed in agency. Does he deliberately invoke her as an icon in humanitarian networks of exchange? Asylum seekers sent to their advocates in Australia, embroideries, small dolls and samplers. These gifts are exchanged in return for the things they need: phone cards, walkmen, cameras, shoes, maps and dictionaries. Many of the objects they request in letters are related to the trade in images and words that sustain them: ways they can capture and communicate their own experience, and sustain connections outside the camp.

Correspondence

These gift exchanges are signs of recognition and ethical responsibility in circumstances where attempts to put a face to an individual asylum seeker were *specifically* proscribed by Australian government policy. It is the young Hazara men held on Nauru who send photographs, and it is this group that is eager to enter into correspondence with Australian activists and use it for a full and frank exchange about their condition. Although the iconic image of the Afghan refugee is a woman, in fact Afghan female asylum seekers on Nauru come into view, veiled and in family group photographs, and few women write letters. When they do, what they have to say is painful. One correspondent, for example, testifies via an amanuensis in letters to Durham and to the Australian minister Philip Ruddock about the specific issues that confront Afghan women: she left Afghanistan with her young daughter following the death of her husband and if she returns, she will be forced to marry her brother-in-law. Other women too, alone on Nauru with young children and no male relatives to act on their behalf as custom requires, testify to their deepening despair and mental illness.

To all intents and purposes, the epistolarium is a cold case and it is now a commodity that has been valued, purchased and archived. And yet, I want to make claims for the letter as an especially potent artifact to capture the spatial, temporal and affective dimensions of the Pacific Solution for both the asylum seekers and their advocates and those of us who read the letters now. What comes together in the relics of the epistolarium are remains of an extraordinary engagement of testimonial exchange: letters in English and in Dari that lack the authentication of singular and consistent handwriting or signature, letters addressed to one correspondent that are taken up by another, photographs and gifts sent to activists by asylum seekers. There are signs of the presence of translators and addressees—those who received these letters in the second person. Envelopes are usually stripped of their stamps; letters marked up in terms of their usefulness for the campaign: publication in newspapers, or a note on when they were read at public meetings, or annotations on whether they might serve for an edited publication of refugee letters; and notes indicate what response was made ('sent batteries', 'sent standard Dari letter'). Sometimes, there is a brief comment on the fate of the refugees 'relocated to New Zealand' or 'returned'. Sometimes, there are copies of letters printed out on recycled papers that are drafts of other correspondence, a quick glimpse of the lives of the activists. These letters are artifacts, unhinged from bodies in space and time, and yet they remain potent. This is especially so when the random exchange of letters coheres into a correspondence and a genuine exchange and engagement is triggered.

The distinction between letters and correspondence determines the organisation of this epistolarium. Stanley distinguishes correspondence as an exchange, as opposed to the single letter. This epistolarium is archived so that, the first boxes contain folders of correspondence, where we have an exchange of letters between a single asylum seeker and one or more Australian recipients, sometimes copies of the reply are included. Then the correspondence peters away to letters: folders of writers represented by fewer than five letters, letters from unidentified asylum seekers (some written in Dari), collective statements jointly authored by asylum seekers and some standard declarations instructing pro bono lawyers to take action on their behalf, forms produced by the 'Spare Rooms for Refugees' activists and completed by asylum seekers who accept offers by Australian volunteers to correspond with them and act as informal guardians in their dealings with government and refugee agencies, newspaper clippings, stamps, patterns for doll-making, sewing and finally, in the last box, fabric bags used for mail. We need to grasp all of these materials and artifacts that comprise this epistolarium, for they speak eloquently of the liminal presence of asylum seekers, their abjection and their agency, and to the intersubjective response of the activists: please forgive us ....

Of all the letters from Nauru, two folders in particular present a fluent correspondence. This is the exchange between the asylum seeker Moh Mehdi, and the activist and addressee Durham, and several other activists.[8] It is Mehdi who can be the most effective translator between the asylum seekers held at Topside and their advocates in Australia: he sends long letters apparently in his own hand, eloquently grasping conditions in the camp, processes of giving testimony to DIMIA, of the long history of oppression of the Hazaras in Afghanistan, and the place of women in Hazara families, and his views on faith and belief. In these letters, the drama and the emotion of life in the camp is grasped vividly and personally. There is a terrible moment in Mehdi's last letter (dated 10/11/02) where he announces he has decided to return to Kabul, he will no longer seek his freedom: 'I don't know how to tell you that I am going back to Afghanistan. I shall be on first flight to Kabul in the next few days. There will be over a hundred people on the plane . . . .'[9]

One of the most eloquent traces of Durham's presence as addressee is incidental and inspired in response to Mehdi. On the reverse of a printed copy of a letter from this most eloquent correspondent, there is a copy of a talk that Durham begins to draft, called 'Profit and Loss in the Pacific':

> Detention letters from Nauru surround me like piles of crumpled leaves, I preserve them as if they're already the past remains or relics of mostly Hazara faces I met in Nauru, a place I'll never forget. The new letters tell me of their bewilderment at the deceits and distortions played upon them in their interviews, in the last rounds, of the last appeals they may ever make.[10]

Mehdi's letters display the signs of *correspondence*: the writer comes alive through a personal and idiosyncratic expression and a direct address to the addressee, and in the letter itself, the handwriting and the signature and the language cohere—he eventually invents an idiosyncratic salutation to begin his letters to Durham; *Dear Madam Kate Durham. Salam Alaikum and G'day.* In this, the Mehdi letters are unusually coherent. By and large, Nauru letters display the difficult labour of their production though inconsistencies: a lined A4 page ripped out of a ring binder, the words transcribed and perhaps falteringly selected from a dictionary, frequent correction of errors, a file apparently from a single correspondent that has no consistency of handwriting or signature to signal individuality and authenticity. It is not unusual to find a page covered in Dari script-perfect lines of filigree in blue biro, to which is attached a translation in crude English. From these, we can only guess what gets lost in translation, and the complex networks around those who testify, their amanuenses and their translators.[11] In all these ways the letters bear the marks of the fact that most asylum seekers are suspended and rendered inarticulate in a legal, linguistic and cultural limbo.

The Gift of Testimony

The letters indicate that, asylum seekers give testimony tactically, and they maneuver as best they can, given in different and contradictory networks simultaneously. This returns me again to intertexts, and an unseen bureaucratic archive that haunts this epistolarium. These Nauru letters are produced at the same time as asylum seekers testify in a series of formal personal interviews with DIMIA—the Australian Department for Immigration, the UNHCR, and the IOM (the International Office for Migration), and their future status depends on the arbitration of these testimonials by these governmental and non-governmental agencies, their institutional addressees. This formal testimony must meet a series of criteria if asylum seekers are to move back into a national community as refugees: authenticity, risk of return, consistency. Few succeed—letters from Nauru repeatedly describe how letters of rejection from DIMIA produce despair on the island, further traumatising a population where the symptoms of post-traumatic stress are already rife. In boxes 3 and 4 we find examples of the formula letter that DIMIA uses to notify asylum seekers that they have been unsuccessful, with appropriate boxes ticked. As always, Moh Mehdi's correspondence includes sharp observations as he reflects on his own failure to qualify for refugee status:

> Currently, every claimant who wishes to seek a review has to participate in counseling sessions in which they tell us the reasons for the rejection. The reasons are sometimes very funny . . . cases rejected for reasons they call discrepancies, inconsistencies, and lack of confidence of the claimants while telling their stories. The fact is that these people seem very poor and powerless against complexities of law and loop-holes for rejection. (14/6/02)

Asylum seekers use letters to activists as supplements, to testify to inconvenient truths that cannot be spoken to DIMIA: Operation Enduring Freedom is not making Afghanistan a safe place for their return, particularly for the Hazara community; the kind of documentation and consistency demanded by the Australian bureaucracy denies the realities of lived experiences of recent Afghan history; they need lawyers and human rights activists on the island to learn appropriate testimony for DIMIA. Letters can appeal to the empathic engagement of the addressee, and they can risk inconsistencies in testimony that must be hidden from DIMIA—benevolent activists read these as signs of authenticity.

The testimonies held in the DIMIA files are a spectral presence that shapes the Nauru letters. Asylum seekers grasp the complex intertextuality between these various narratives, and what constitutes appropriate memory, experience, subjectivity and agency for the various addressees of their testimony. Yet they also narrate out of a condition where they are unknown to themselves, where their assigned number and the name of their ship mark a new emergent subjectivity and identity as asylum seekers, perpetually adrift from home, family, tradition, profession and suspended in time and place. Nauru letters grasp this implicitly: in the faltering, broken expression and content of individual letters (where they often comment on their inability to continue to write/speak); in the random inexplicable termination of lines of correspondence. There is nothing conclusive in the epistolarium, and this is entirely appropriate and, in fact, authentic. As artifact, the Nauru letter remains faithful to its origins in the deliberate alienation of asylum seekers from human society, and their struggle to gain entry into a free and democratic community.

All of this gives an extraordinary resonance to that idea of the letter as a theatre for the performance of the self, for the Nauru asylum seekers the deliberate policy of dehumanising and bestialising the other becomes a lived experience realised in the space and time of their incarceration. The theatrical metaphor would not surprise the first person correspondents. We see in this archive how asylum seekers maneuver to give testimony in quite different circuits synchronically, and their lives hang upon the power of their testimony to get the address right in each case. There is an uncanny incarnation between these letters and their first person: these are bodies in limbo—suspended in air, as Bowman Ali tells us. These letters are apocalyptic; they emerge from the end of the world and they struggle to testify to the birth of a new self-silenced and demonised in a terrible condition of statelessness. The letters reveal the shape of a collective memory emerging on the Nauru, as the community of asylum seekers narrate not just the trauma of persecution and violence in Afghanistan, but bruising encounters with the military forces and bureaucracy of a nation that is, in theory, a passionate advocate of human rights.

It is the language of human rights discourse, an established protocol and ethics for cross-cultural engagement, that shapes the rhetoric of Nauru letters.[12] Although some critics (Brant) suggest that letters *prove* we are human, Nauru letters speak from a condition where this recognition is not secured. They deliberately challenge stereotypes of asylum seekers as terrorists, aliens, and uncaring parents (the children overboard affair). A delicate transaction occurs: in this tradition of human rights activism, both the letter writer and the addressee, the first and the second person, are humanised and equalised in the process of writing and receiving letters in recognition and empathic engagement. This reciprocity is tenuous and must be constantly and carefully sustained. Asylum seekers have no doubts that the status of the human is an identity as precarious as any other, to be carefully and tactically acquired and nurtured at all costs.

Stanley has suggested that, Marcel Mauss's work on the gift is useful for grasping the economy of epistolary exchanges. As I have argued elsewhere, gifting is particularly appropriate to grasp the currency of testimony (Whitlock, 2004). Nauru letters figure this exchange explicitly: asylum seekers request goods, and sometimes precisely: a 'good' watch, Adidas trainers, a clipping of an image of a Sony walkman plus cassettes. Activists respond as best as they can; sometimes apologetically: a watch is possible but not a 'good' watch, the requests are so many they cannot be fulfilled and, sometimes, more critically: so many cameras have been sent and few images returned. Tactics are omnipresent in this epistolary economy: asylum seekers make requests of privileged Australian citizens in exchange for their testimony which is one of the few commodities they have to offer, and in return, activists harvest from letters the fragments of testimony that might be used in human rights advocacy and benevolence on their behalf. Gifting through testimony entails an economy of the emotions and affect: Mehdi reminds of the emotional costs of representing trauma for asylum seekers, and activist expiate their guilt and anger at what is done in their name as Australian citizens; their activism humanises both the asylum seekers and themselves as citizens of a globalised world.[13] In fact, the project of humanising Australian citizens remains a recurring rationale for the ongoing circulation of asylum seeker stories.[14]

The Epistolary Triad

Clearly the production and reception of Nauru letters is a crowded scene. Testimony seeks out to those who will bear witness, and these letters allow intricate negotiations of recognition and response between the first person, those who give witness, and the second person—the addressee who responds in recognition. I enter this epistolarium belatedly, translating it in terms of a different place and time when the letter writer, translators and recipients have departed the stage. But, it remains emotionally charged nevertheless. As autobiographical artifacts, Nauru letters are at the centre of a dense and ongoing series of relations in the production and transmission of trauma narrative. Stanley turns to Mikhail Bakhtin's observation that, 'There are always (at least) two sides to any correspondence ... Indeed, the situation is even more complicated, for ... the public nature of epistolary writing should also alert us to traces of the third-person reader outside the traditional epistolary dyad' (100). The epistolarium becomes even more crowded at this point, then. As I have suggested, we see signs of many hands, tongues and ears in the production of Nauru letters in the detention centre in the work of those who testify, their translators and amanuenses; there is rarely a singular first person 'writer' in this epistolarium. Equally, the addressee of Nauru letters is multiple. The second person, conventionally understood as the addressee, is not private or singular. The activists respond to Nauru letters individually, but the letters are forwarded to others if they appear to offer important or particularly worrying evidence of abuse, they are read aloud at public meetings, they are incorporated variously into an active campaign on behalf of the asylum seekers. In the case of Nauru letters, we need to think of this 'third person' that gives 'meaning and shape and form' (Stanley 101) to the collection: the reader who enters the epistolarium as a belated reader and witness.

Here the mutual metonymy that Stanley suggests is triggered by the letter places both second and third person recipients in a position of terrible responsibility as witnesses to trauma story that continues to circle and carry affective force. We can see this played out around Nauru letters in an array of multimedia epitexts that extend beyond these immediate boxed artifacts and are the work of witnessing in the second and third person. Firstly, there are the extracts of letters from Australian detention centres (including Nauru) included in the edition called *From Nowhere to Zero*, edited by Janet Austin, published in

2003. Secondly, the BBC documentary made by Durham and the British journalist Sarah Macdonald captured images of the Nauru detention centres and was screened in the UK in 2002. Thirdly, there is the vast collection of artwork that was made by Durham—286 works of art that are the testimony of the addressee, the recipient who is haunted by what she hears from the asylum seekers. These are now part of the Fryer epistolarium. Fourthly and finally, there is the scholarly work that now proceeds from this archived collection, the work of the third person.

The epistolarium becomes vast and busy at this point: it includes all the images and texts that get bound up with it, the letters and photographs and objects that are sent from Nauru, and the responses of the second and third person recipients who become caught in the ongoing effects of testimony. In the case of the Nauru epistolarium, there is an extraordinary representation of all this: a series of artworks by the addressee, a figuration of that mutual metonymy that Stanley talks about. Durham is an emotional centre of this multimedia archive as its most powerful addressee, and the extraordinary proliferation of her art work inspired, or should I say *haunted,* by witnessing trauma is in itself an eloquent expression of the affective force of the letters. Let me speculate about some further signs that connect this art work to the letter, to suggest how Durham has figured here a response that translates and figures her role as the addressee of numerous letters from Nauru.

The Artist as Second Person

The Burnside/Durham collection includes 272 painted panels, oil on composition board, each 20 cm × 20 cm, which forms three works collectively titled SIEV.X. These images were first displayed at an exhibition on 20 November 2004, and a selection can now be viewed at Durham's 'artwork' archive online.[15] Durham's paintings are haunted by the terrible stories of the Pacific crossing that recur time and again in Nauru letters. Attempts to gain access to the Australian mainland which (as Moh Mehdi writes in his letter) was thought of as a place of light and freedom after the darkness and brutality of Afghanistan were traumatic and, in the case of SIEV X, fatal.[16]. The crossing remains with the asylum seekers in traumatic memory and in identity, incorporated into their rebirth and identification as detainees—in fact images of drowning recur across the letters, and the names of ships such as Tobruk, Manoora and Tampa become part of the classification system on Nauru that is taken up subjectively in letters.

The multiple small panels are the signature work of the artwork of this Nauru epistolarium, and the association of the collage, the numerous small portraits and the letter is indicative. Durham features the careful individuation of asylum seekers which was specifically proscribed by Australian government policy, and which emerges in the intimate and direct address of the Nauru letters, caught in individual frames of death by drowning. These 20 cm square pictures were replicated as postcards[17], and a selected series of images from the original exhibition appears in a virtual gallery.[18] But in the real gallery, these small frames are then gathered together in an overwhelming installation and a structure of steel framed display panels, 180 cm × 90 cm, that is also part of the archive. This installation gathers the individual panels into a collage that amplifies and connects these individual frames of traumatic death and confronts the viewer with the apocalyptic experience that haunts the asylum seekers. Here we find a correlation or perhaps an oscillation between the individual and the collective, and I am reminded of Stanley's comments on the ways that letters can refract back and forth across other representational versions of a life 'thereby piecing together a kaleidoscopic image of them' (224) Durham is the emotional epicenter, the addressee of many Nauru letters, and between 2002 and 2004 she produced an extraordinary number of art works that not only represent the traumatic experiences of the asylum seeker but also speak back to, or perhaps speak of, the letter as fragment of trauma story that remains embedded in the second person witness.

In the Third Person

Nauru letters grasp the extraordinary perverse dynamics of post 9/11 border panic, and the spectral presence of asylum seekers continues to haunt those of us who encounter the epistolarium now and witness the suffering of asylum seekers anew. Librarians and other researchers often come and look at the letters as they surround me in the library as one of its recent acquisitions. We share relief that one of the first acts of the new Rudd government was to end the Pacific Solution and close the Nauru detention facility. These letters remain alive, and are potent triggers of shame. How we enter and engage with the traumatic narratives in this epistolarium now, as a belated third person, is an important issue. There is the risk of a distinctly contemporary logic: this archive of letters and effects is now available to us just in time to enter into a narrative of national renewal, as if the disbanding of the Pacific Solution and the demise of the Howard government removes a temporary aberration. In her recent discussion of the film about asylum seekers, *Finding Ali*, Bernadette Brennan speculates that future generations will find the mandatory detention system as incomprehensible as we now find the White Australia policy. Others fear is all too comprehensible: 'in our treatment of them—desperate, defenceless, and traumatized—we identify something of our character...'(Burnside 124).

Letters, perhaps more than any other artifact reminds us of the uniqueness of life narrative: the difference between life narrative and other forms of historical record is the performance of rhetorical acts: the justification of subjective perceptions, disputing alternative accounts, conveying cultural information with subjective force, an active and persuasive engagement with the witness. In the letter, these rhetorical elements of assertion, justification, judgement and interrogation assume an intimate and personal force that produce powerful affects of shame, complicity and responsibility. This is the legacy of the Nauru letters. We rarely enter into correspondence with Afghan refugees, when we do, we find an intimate and painful insight into the limitations of human rights discourse, and the continuing drive of paranoid nationalism in the making of Australian citizenship.

Notes

[1] Working with these letters raises a number of ethical issues, and one of these is whether asylum seekers should be recognised by name. I have used initials unless the correspondents are identified elsewhere (for example Mohammed Mehdi is identified at Kate Durham's website) or where I have explicit permission. References are to the date of the correspondence. I acknowledge with thanks Bowman Ali's permission to use his photograph and to quote from his correspondence, by personal communication, July 2008.

[2] Beyond the attacks on New York and Washington, there is the war in Iraq, terrorist attacks in Europe Africa and the Middle East, the war in Afghanistan, the carceral archipelago of deterritorialised spaces of containment that stretched from Guantanamo to the central Pacific, and the ongoing surges of dispossessed people from the Middle and Far East.

[3] The 1984 and 2001 images of Sharbat Gula and the story of her return can be viewed online at the National Geographic photo gallery: http://ngm.nationalgeographic.com/2002/04/afghan-girl/index-text. It is also the subject of a documentary screened periodically on the Discovery channel. See too the discussion of this image in the Introduction to Hesford and Kozol and Whitlock.

[4] AA writes on 14/7/03: The other IOM personals are from Australian pushton sects They have not forgotten their ancient enemies to us Hazaras. Even in the camp they have not spared their fanaticism and spite. Every sort of persecution which is possible they are imposing on refugees. On 18/10/03 All interpreters here are sunni believers or they are from puston or tajick sects. They are not compassionate, have enmity with Hazaras and shia believers.

[5] 24/3/03 from JR (in Melbourne) to asylum seeker EH: 'I am ashamed as are hundreds and thousands of my fellow Australians that JH has committed us to this abominable war created by the USA. Stay as healthy as you can. No one can force you to return to Afg. You are safe.' 15/08/02 from JR (in Melbourne) to AS: 15/08/02: 'From Jenny: please write to us and try to forgive our country.'

[6] New Zealand took over 400 asylum seekers from Australia's offshore processing centres, and sent teams to Afghanistan, Iraq, Pakistan and Iran to track down the families of refugees and offer them permanent resettlement. (Gordon 42)

[7] These letters were exchanged alongside other communications that leave fewer 'hard' traces, see for example Kate Douglas's analysis of email correspondence with asylum seekers.

[8] Kate Durham speaks of this correspondence with her friend Mohammed at her website, and given this I include his proper name here, as filed in the Fryer collection.

[9] As David Corlett remarks in his study of returned asylum seekers, many of those who returned feared their loss of humanity due to the terrible slow psychological disintegration resulting from indefinite detention. See too Moorhead's chapter on returned refugees and asylum seekers.

[10] A version of this can now be read at Durham's website.

[11] N.d. MNA (Folder 4, Box 1) 3 pages of Dari script reduced to list: no electricity, candles, water too hot, weather too hot, need cold water.

[12] 1/6/02. MAA: 'we are drowning in this wave of Australian politics ... Where are those humanitarian organisations that defend human rights? And where are those humanitarian slogans? There's nobody to hear our voice, to listen to us, to defend out rights. I remember the day when I read in a magazine that a car was trapped in a tunnel in a Western country, and that they spend thousands of dollars to rescue it. But today, I think we refugees do not even have the value of that cat ... we spent thousands of US dollars in order to live like a human being ... Why do they not think of us as equals?'

[13] Klaus Neumann argues that, whereas the hardline policy of the Pacific Solution was not unprecedented in Australia, the humanitarian commitment and responsibility felt by individuals as citizens of a globalised world was unprecedented.

[14] See, for example, Bernadette Brennan's discussion of Clara Law's film 'Letter to Ali', the introductions to anthologies such as Austin and Leach and Mansouri, among others, and Gordon's study of one specific asylum seeker held on Nauru, *Freeing Ali: The Human Face of the Pacific Solution*.

[15] http://www.katedurham.com/03_ss/index.asp?g_id = 1

[16] In October 2001, a boat carrying about 400 asylum seekers set out for Australia from Indonesia, and entered the surveillance zone of Australian coastal defence operations, identified as SIEV X. It was grossly overloaded and sank, almost all the people on board, mostly women and children, drowned. An archive of resources about SIEV X are available at http://www.safecom.org.au/canberra07-sievx.htm

[17] See http://www.katedurham.com/03_ss/slide.asp?c_slideshow_id = 1.

[18] See http://www.katedurham.com/03_ss/slide.asp?c_slideshow_id = 3.

References

Austin, Janet. *From Nothing to Zero: Letters from Refugees in Australia's Detention Centres*. Melbourne: Lonely Planet, 2003.

Brennan, Bernadette. *'Travelling towards ourselves: Rights and recognition in Clara Law's 'Letters to Ali''*. Ed. Bernadette Brennan. Just Words. Australian Authors Writing for Justice. St. Lucia: U of Queensland P, 2008. 137–57.

Burnside, Julian. *Watching Brief. Reflection on Human Rights, Law, and Justice*. Melbourne, Austral.: Scribe, 2007.

Butler, Judith. *Precarious Life: The Powers of Mourning and Violence*. London: Verso, 2004.

Corlett, David. *Following Them Home. The Fate of the Returned Asylum Seekers*. Melbourne, Austral.: Black Inc., 2005.

Douglas, Kate. 'Witnessing on the Web: Asylum Seekers and Letter-Writing Projects on Australian Activist Websites.' a/b. *Auto/Biography Studies* 21.1 (Summer 2006): 44–57.

Gordon, Michael. *Freeing Ali: The Human Face of the Pacific Solution*. Sydney, Austral.: UNSW Press, 2005.

Gregory, Derek. *The Colonial Present. Afghanistan, Palestine, Iraq*. Malden, MA: Blackwell Publishing, 2004.

Hesford, Wendy S., and Wendy Kozol. *Just Advocacy? Women's Human Rights, Transnational Feminisms, and the Politics of Representation*. New Brunswick NJ: Rutgers UP, 2005.

Jolly, Margaretta. 'Introduction: Epistolarity in the Twenty-First Century.' a/b. *Auto/Biography Studies* 21.1 (Summer 2006): 1–6.

Jolly, Margaretta, and Liz Stanley. 'Letters as/not a genre.' *Life Writing* 2.2 (Jan. 2005): 91–118.

katedurham.com. 6 Aug. 2008. <http://www.katedurham.com>.

Leach, Michael and Fethi Mansouri. *Lives in Limbo: Voices of Refugees Under Temporary Protection*. Sydney, Austral.: UNSW Press, 2004.

Moorhead, Caroline. *Human Cargo. A Journey Among Refugees*. London: Vintage, 2006.

Neumann, Klaus. Refuge Australia. *Australia's Humanitarian Record*. Sydney, Austral.: UNSW Press, 2004.

Sontag, Susan. *Regarding the Pain of Others*. London: Hamish Hamilton, 2003.

Stanley, Liz. 'The epistolarium: on theorizing letters and correspondences.' *Auto/Biography* 12 (2004): 201–35.

Whitlock, Gillian. *Soft Weapons: Autobiography in Transit*. Chicago: U of Chicago P, 2007.

Whittlock, Gillian. (2004) Consuming Passions: Reconciliation in women's, intellectual memoir, *Tulsa Studies in Women's Literature*, 23(1): 13–28.

Hostile Witness: Torture Testimony in the War on Terror

Nina Philadelphoff-Puren

In J. M. Coetzee's novel *Waiting for the Barbarians*, the local magistrate—'a civil servant with literary ambitions' (169)—receives the disturbing Colonel Joll into the colony to conduct interrogations. Sympathetically imagining himself into the position of the prisoners and anxious to understand their predicament, the magistrate draws the Colonel into conversation. 'What if your prisoner is telling the truth,' he asks, 'yet finds he is not believed? Is that not a terrible position?' The Colonel dismisses the magistrate's concerns with an explanation of his scientific procedure for distinguishing true statements from false ones: 'First I get lies, you see—this is what happens—first lies, then pressure, then more lies, then more pressure, then the break, then more pressure, then the truth. This is how you get the truth' (5). The Colonel's performative description invokes the process of torture itself, with its excruciating repetitions and its fondness for euphemism: not pain, but 'pressure'; not torture, just a way of extracting 'the truth'. In depicting torture in this way, the Colonel invokes its ancient predicates: that torture cleanly targets the prisoner in possession of certain words; that truthful words only emerge after the 'touchstone' (duBois 7) of torture has been pressed to their body; and that without such pain, the prisoner's words cannot be trusted.

Coetzee's eerily prescient novel anticipates the structures of justification that underlie the practice of torture in the War on Terror: Guantanamo Bay houses 'bad men' in possession of critical information, and 'alternative interrogation procedures' such as water-boarding are required to bring this information to light (Office of the Press Secretary). These premises, repeated *ad nauseum*, have created a normative framework in which detainee speech is configured as fundamentally untruthful unless both extracted and verified by the procedures of so-called coercion. It follows from this model that those words produced outside of interrogation—words that might, for example, refer to the process of interrogation itself, by renaming it torture—are subject to doubt.

As I will show below in relation to the torture testimony of two Australian citizens—Mamdouh Habib and David Hicks—this narrative arrangement produces a case of 'inexpressibility' as recently described by Darius Rejali (2007). In a reorientation of Elaine Scarry's (1985) influential account of the language-destroying power of torture, Rejali argues that 'the inexpressibility that matters in torture is the gap between speakers and their communities, not the brain and the tongue' (580). This claim recasts the linguistic problem of torture from the scene of the interrogator's cell—in which the detainee's power to produce a signifying narrative is annihilated through the administration of pain—to the public sphere in which the detainee who has survived torture attests to what has been done to them. Inexpressibility in this context thus means not that the detainee 'cannot utter' the testimony, but rather that having uttered it, it somehow fails profoundly to take effect, to be taken *up* by the political community to whom it is addressed. I argue that this testimonial intransitivity is the result of at least three entwined phenomena: the normative narrative frameworks of the War on Terror which consign testimony about torture to the domain of the unspeakable (Butler *Excitable* 133); the operation of what I will call here 'the hostile witness', a form of the second person committed to discrediting rather than enabling traumatic narratives; and a generalised attack on detainees' ability to narrate (Slaughter) which is evident at the level of rhetoric and law.

The experience of Mamdouh Habib and David Hicks dramatises the painful human consequences of the 'inexpressibility' of torture testimony in the War on Terror. Profoundly disruptive of the Australian government's hagiographic narration of American power. This testimony has languished on the borders of public debate, widely known but not yet independently investigated. Mamdouh Habib was arrested in Pakistan in October 2001, then interrogated in Pakistan, Egypt and Guantanamo Bay. He registered complaints of torture in each location from mid-2002, in letters to his family and reports to the Red Cross and Australian government officials (Forbes and Debelle). Released without charge back to Australia in January 2005, Habib immediately took possession of his story. He presented his narrative of extraordinary rendition and torture on high-rating current affairs programs and gave speeches at universities around the country. Controversially, he reported that, Australian officials were involved in his detention and interrogation, a claim that is now the subject of a major litigation before the Federal Court of NSW (McClymont). From the first, however, numerous attempts were made to both physically silence him and discredit his words. Government officials attempted to both obstruct his public appearances and impugn his character, while unknown assailants threatened to kill him should he continue to speak out. Despite the seriousness of his claims, there has to date been no independent inquiry into his case, and there has been limited public interest in his story.[1]

David Hicks's testimony about torture has been similarly left in limbo, despite his ultimately extraordinary public profile in Australia. Hicks was arrested by the Northern Alliance in December 2001, and then handed to the US Military. He was detained for more than six years without charge in Guantanamo Bay, a period that includes one of the longest periods of sensory deprivation on the CIA's record books (McCoy 25). Labelled a 'terrorist' from the first stages of his confinement, Hicks was effectively abandoned by the Australian government, which repeatedly insisted that the United States had the right to treat him as it saw fit—even if that treatment included indefinite detention without trial (Mitchell). Importantly, while Hicks's case attracted little interest in Australia for the first four years, public opinion changed rapidly after the US Supreme Court in Hamdan ruled that the Military Commission process (which had charged Hicks) was unconstitutional. After this point, Hicks became a growing domestic political issue (Stewart). By the time of his controversial plea bargain in February 2007, he was the subject of an incendiary public debate, with numerous actions groups, peak legal bodies and church leaders calling almost daily for him to be immediately returned to Australia. Despite this extraordinary public attention—which even threatened the election chances of the incumbent conservative Howard government—Hicks's torture allegations never succeeded in coming completely into focus. Like Habib, Hicks complained to Australian officials about his treatment in mid-2002 (Forbes and Debelle), before producing two further affidavits that documented a litany of human rights violations. In the first of these narratives (which was publicly released in December 2004), Hicks describes being injected with unknown substances, and subjected to mock executions, sleep deprivation and solitary confinement (Hicks 'Affidavit'). The Australian government cast doubt on these claims and refused to independently examine them, instead charging US authorities with this responsibility (AAP 'Ruddock'). The second affidavit was produced in February 2007, at the same time as Hicks was negotiating a controversial plea bargain which would bring his confinement to a close (Allard). The peculiar requirements of this plea bargain (which I will discuss later in this article) required Hicks to repudiate all of his previous claims about torture. This 'agreement' ostensibly dispatched Hicks's detailed allegations about torture with a single sentence, without any further institutional process inquiring into their validity. As a result, David Hicks's torture testimony has never been independently examined nor formally answered.

As Kay Schaffer and Sidonie Smith have argued, the circulation of narratives about human rights violations can galvanise political communities into establishing institutional procedures of verification, exposure and reparation (3). The Canadian investigation into the torture claims of Maher Arar is a case in point: this inquiry resulted in the official acknowledgement of Arar's testimony of extraordinary rendition and torture at the hands of US officials, and significant compensation and an apology (CBC News). However, the torture testimony of Mamdouh Habib and David Hicks has so far failed to produce similar political emotions in its audience, despite Australia being, like Canada, a liberal democracy with a strong tradition of defending and advocating the values of human rights discourse, at least until recently.[2] Despite Mamdouh Habib's repeated public presentations of his traumatic narrative, and the exceptional community interest in the prolonged incarceration of David Hicks, the torture testimony of these men remains consigned to the shadowy interval between knowledge and acknowledgement described by Thomas Nagel (1998)—widely publicised, certainly, but never formally tested, adjudicated and answered in an institutional forum.

At least in part, this can be attributed to the powerful challenge that such testimony presents to the hegemonic narrative of the War on Terror which controls the form and terms of public debate in Australia. As Judith Butler explains 'In the United States, we begin the story by invoking a first-person narrative point of view, and telling what happened on September 11' (*Precarious Life* 5). In the story of 'what happened', the United States figures as an injured 'I', the passive and unimplicated victim of unthinkable violence. To question the frame of this narration—to suggest it may in fact begin at another point, and be focalised through the perspective of different protagonists—has been to risk the charge of moral equivocation and an alignment with the perpetrators (2). Torture testimony disrupts the seamless operation of this narrative from another direction. Such testimony challenges the unequivocal victim status of the injured American 'I', and instead recasts that 'I' itself into the position of the perpetrator of unthinkable acts. As well as casting the United States as the agent of violence, such testimony also claims for its speaker the moral authority of one who has suffered a human rights violation. In this way, such witnessing contests the ordering of the dominant narrative, in which the only 'legitimate' victim in the War on Terror is America and its citizens (Bennet 179).

The inadmissibility of the phrase 'American torturer' in the mediascapes (Appadurai 37) of Australian public discourse was demonstrated by the former Australian Foreign Minister Alexander Downer in February 2005, when he was asked to comment on Mamdouh Habib's appearance on the popular *60 Minutes* program shortly after his release without charge from Guantanamo Bay. In a remarkable interview, Habib had provided a detailed account of his experiences of torture while detained as a terror suspect in Egypt and later in Guantanamo Bay ('Under Suspicion'). Asked whether he found Habib's testimony convincing, the Foreign Minister remarked: 'You can weigh up in relation to the allegations of torture whether you believe a man who has allegedly been involved with

Al Qaeda, or whether you believe the Americans. It depends on where your prejudice lies, I suppose' (Downer). Mr Downer here invokes the coercive false dichotomy that structures the broader narrative of the War on Terror: 'Either you are with us or you are with the terrorists' (qtd. in Moeller 63), in order to control the possible interpretations of Mamdouh Habib's dangerous words about torture. In this passage, Mr Downer not only impugns Habib's testimony, but also issues a veiled threat to the citizen-subject who might listen to him. To attend to the one who invokes the illegitimate phrasing of 'American torturer' is to oneself risk alignment with 'terrorists' in the over-arching narrative structure. Such a move has a regulative effect on the shape of the public debate about torture, and the positions that are available for those who have witnessed such testimony and seek to respond. As Judith Butler explains 'dissent is quelled, in part, through threatening the speaking subject with an uninhabitable identification. Because it would be heinous to identify as treasonous, as a collaborator, one fails to speak, or speaks in throttled ways, in order to sidestep the terrorising identification that threatens to take hold' (*Precarious Life* xix). Mr Downer's response to Mamdouh Habib is not just one possible move in a field of heteroglossia, but rather is designed to itself determine what could constitute a 'reasonable' response to his narrative. In simple terms, Mr Downer's words foreclose the possibility that a citizen could interpret Habib's testimony in a positive light, or decide that his testimony justified a call for institutional scrutiny or indeed a Royal Commission.[3] Instead, Mr Downer restricts the scope of the critical debate by aligning belief in Habib's words with support for terrorism.

The regulatory control exercised over the possible meanings of torture testimony in Australia is in part enabled through the politics of genre that governs its presentation. As an Australian senator remarked in a parliamentary discussion of the torture and rendition of Mamdouh Habib, 'like most Australians, my knowledge of this issue has come to me through the newspapers' (Legal and Constitutional Committee). In the mediascapes of the War on Terror, torture testimony is conventionally presented in the highly mediated format of hard news reporting (although there are also important items testimony published on the internet).[4] In this respect, the performance of this testimony is intimately linked to the rules of the genre in which it appears. Hard news reporting in both print and television requires journalists to canvas the counter-case and alternative views (White 216). Because the torture allegations of Mamdouh Habib and David Hicks implicate government officials and Australia's relationship with the United States, such officials are regularly called upon to 'respond' to the testimony within the same textual frame as its performance. But, this genre rule has invidious consequences in the case of the reporting of human rights violations like torture. The discourse of 'balance' elides the fact that the contemporary mediascape is not a democratic agon inhabited by equivalently positioned subjects, each in possession of words of similar force. When a terror suspect speaks of torture from Guantanamo Bay and is 'answered' by a government official, that speech itself will be an object of conflict in a field riven by systems of domination (Foucault) in which the suspect's words are all too easily disqualified.

The generic convention of 'official comment' has important consequences for the way in which torture testimony is both staged and interpreted. Picked up and re-cited in contexts far away from the original act of speaking (in which, for example, a human rights lawyer or activist was the immediate addressee), such testimony is then reiterated through multiple channels of news media reporting, which proliferate new scenes of address for this testimony and critically establish government officials in the privileged role of 'second person': that is, the recipient of the testimony and its witness (Whitlock 'Second Person'). However, the operation of the 'second person' in these instances diverges from traditional accounts of the ideal role and function of such a figure in the testimonial exchange. In Shoshana Felman and Dori Laub's influential account of ethical witnessing, the 'second person' enters a state of ecstatic identification in which they are pollinated by the affect and the narrative of the one testifying, thus partially experiencing the trauma themselves (37). Intensely grounded in a face-to-face encounter between the first and second person, this ecstatic model of listening obscures the *textuality* of the process of 'witnessing' a reported narrative of an event; it belies the fact that, testimony and its witnessing can in fact give rise to a struggle over words, a battle of linguistic and rhetorical acts, particularly when the narrative disrupts and indeed contests the rules of the dominant social story in which the testimony takes its place. When traumatic narratives give rise to (social and political) antagonism rather than empathic identification, the second person operates in a different ethical modality to the 'blank screen' of Laub's description (37). Instead of working to deliver the testimony into ratified circuits of deliberation, such a witness instead strives to consign it to the domain of the 'inexpressible' by impugning both the words and the character of the one testifying. As Joseph Slaughter has argued, human rights violations attack the subject's powers of narration; the second person in this model is thus a *rhetorical* adjunct to the physical and psychological violations against detainees that are now so copiously documented (Rose; Stafford Smith; and Thompson and Paglen).

Such a person might be usefully described as a 'hostile witness', and it is the work of this figure that is in part responsible for the failure of torture testimony in Australia to gain both critical and moral purchase in the community. The citizen-viewer consumes not just the narrative of a human rights violation in a hard news report, but also the co-terminous scene of its vanquishment. For example, in an interview in May 2004, the former Australian Prime Minister, Mr John Howard, was asked to comment on the news that an eye-witness had reported seeing David Hicks tied up and beaten by US forces in Afghanistan (Grimshaw). In his reply, the Prime Minister chose to reflect on the torture allegations of both David Hicks and Mamdouh Habib. He remarked, 'I find it strange that these allegations of abuse against Mr Hicks and Mr Habib have arisen only since the prisoner abuse scandal erupted in relation to the American forces.' This observation was founded on a fiction: Mamdouh Habib and David Hicks in fact informed Australian officials that they had been abused as early as May 2002, but only those citizens particularly familiar with these cases would be aware of this discrepancy (Forbes and Debelle). Having tendentiously edited the record of notification in this way, the Prime Minister then uses the Abu Ghraib prison scandal to undermine Hicks and Habib's claims to have been tortured. The Prime Minister's words suggest that any allegations which emerge after that scandal can only be a suspicious and illegitimate copy of the original Abu Ghraib complaints. Perversely, the very visibility and ubiquity of the Abu Ghraib images is made to establish that subsequent torture testimony is *less* likely rather than more likely to be true. As the Prime Minister concludes, 'We do have to place that caveat and take these allegations with a grain of salt.' In the absence of an independent inquiry into such testimony, this staged antagonistic 'dialogue' becomes a defacto adjudication of the testimony's legitimacy. In this way, the circulation and transmission of media reports of human rights violations constitute a kind of 'dangerous supplement' (Derrida *Grammatology*) to the juridical process that has itself still not taken place.

The work of the hostile witness is facilitated by the particular features of torture in the War on Terror, and their relationship to forensic narrative. The detainee testimony recorded so far conforms to a distinct pattern. As is now well known, detainees describe being subject to painful stress positions and hooding; sleep deprivation and solitary confinement; loud noises and extremes of temperature.[5] These practices are sometimes described as 'torture-lite' or 'clean-torture' (Rejali 4). Such tactics are particularly cruel because they eschew the employment of complex torture equipment and instead turn the prisoner's own body and character into the instruments of pain. In stress positions, it is the prisoner's own tissue and blood vessels which violently expand, causing excruciating suffering in the various forms of humiliation. It is one's own character that is the target of power as the protocols of torture coercively construct the prisoner as a certain kind of subject (Butler 'Sexual Politics').

Moreover, such techniques are able to exploit a kind of 'plausible deniability' with their apparently anodyne nature: witness Donald Rumsfeld's famous handwritten note objecting that, detainees should only be forced to stand for four hours at a time: '... I stand for 8-hours a day', he scoffed, a remark which analogises the excruciating torture of forced standing while indefinitely detained to the unremarkable practice of writing freely at a lectern (Haynes). In Australia, the former Attorney-General Philip Ruddock similarly disputed whether sleep deprivation (as suffered by David Hicks) should properly be designated a human rights violation. 'I don't regard sleep deprivation as torture. I've not heard it being put that way' (AAP 'Sleep Deprivation'). In each case, the absence of explicit instruments of torture is able to contribute to the argument that torture itself was not taking place.

But even more critically, so-called 'clean torture' appears to have found favour in democratic societies like the United States because, it ostensibly 'leaves no marks' on the bodies of the prisoners who suffer it. Darius Rejali argues that because extensive public monitoring is a feature of such societies, torture techniques that apparently leave no trace enable officials to avoid 'the crises of legitimacy' that would ensue should the practice of torture actually be exposed (9). But why should a form of torture that leaves no marks enable the regimes that employ it to evade detection in this way? Would we not still have the detainee's words about the event? The problem here is the relationship between evidence, injury and narration. As Rejali explains, 'allegations of torture are simply less credible when there is nothing to show for it. In the absence of visible wounds or photographs of actual torture, who is one to believe?' (8) Without the verifying power of forensic evidence, narrative testimony about torture enters a contest of claim and counter-claim that terror suspects are poorly positioned to win. In his appearance on the *60 Minutes* program, Mamdouh Habib reported that he had confessed to a series of terrorist acts—such as training the pilots of the planes that flew into the World Trade Centre, and moving chemicals in Afghanistan—only because he was being tortured. 'I have nothing true,' he said, 'I make him happy. I want to save myself' ('Under Suspicion'). Asked to comment on this testimony the following day, the then Foreign Minister Alexander Downer remarked that, 'remember, we have no evidence except his own claims—the claims of somebody who allegedly has been involved with Al Qaeda—that he was subjected to torture' (Downer). The Minister here exploits the gap between evidence and narration to again construct a coercive interpretative consensus on what Habib's testimony about torture can be understood to mean: all we have are his words, and here they are subject to doubt.

But narrative testimony alone is not the only target here—the Minister's response also regulates who will and will not count as a viable speaking subject (Butler *Excitable Speech* 136) in the context of torture. On the Minister's model, 'somebody who has been involved with Al Qaeda' simple cannot produce legitimate or even testable words. Rhetorically, this strategy draws on a long tradition of techniques which have as their aim the discrediting of torture testimony. In John Conroy's study of the British government's reaction to the revelations that, they were torturing Northern Irish prisoners in the early 1970s, it was shown that discrediting can take a number of forms, including denial and minimisation (230–32). Such moves would be familiar to observers of the unfolding narrative of the Abu Ghraib prison scandal, in which the Bush Administration went from denying that human rights violations were taking place (prior to the release of the photographs), to reframing the scandal from a question of torture to a question of abuse.[6] However, the principal strategy in any program of disqualification is the wholesale discrediting of the one testifying. In Aristotelian rhetoric, the establishment of *ethos* is one of the principal methods of conducting a persuasive argument, and likewise an attack on *ethos* is a potent way to undermine and cast doubt on the speaker's claims. An efficient way to do this is to apply an 'uninhabitable' appellation to the speaker, such as the term 'terrorist'.[7]

While this term has a complex discursive history (Porras), in its current formation, it is overwhelmingly associated with the attacks on the World Trade

Centre and the Pentagon on 11 September 2001. In the dominant ideoscapes of the War on Terror, the 'terrorist' is beyond the purview of rational sympathy, with the designation marking the limits of the human itself and depriving the subject of the cover and protection of international law (Butler *Precarious Life* xvi). But the term itself is afflicted by a fatal conceptual vagueness. The Department of Defence's own data (Denbeaux and Denbeauz) illustrates the exceptionally broad and spurious criteria used to designate so-called 'enemy combatants' or 'Taliban supporters' in Guantanamo Bay (both terms synonyms for 'terrorist' in the solecistic narrative structures of the War on Terror). For example, one could be designated as 'an enemy combatant' simply for being in possession of a Casio watch or wearing drab olive clothing (17); one could be termed a 'Taliban supporter' even when conscripted into their forces as a minor (16). The looseness and incoherence of the criteria here is amplified by the subsequent lack of distinction that is made between persons. As Seymour Hersh has remarked in relation to those detained in Guantanamo Bay, 'there's absolutely no differentiation among those who are people who wanted to do something, conspired against America or were Al Qaeda members, and those who are simply caught up in the American sweeps. There is no differentiation' (2). Indeed, in December 2006, the then Guantanamo Bay commander stated of the men who were then currently detained, 'They're all terrorists, all enemy combatants. I don't think there's such a thing as a medium security terrorist' (Golden). At the time of this comment, not one of the men so described had been charged with a single crime, and scores have been released without charge in the intervening period.

In these contexts, it is clear that the appellation 'terrorist' (and its synonyms) is functioning non-juridically; that is, it is not applied to persons subject to formal legal processes of identification and prosecution. Indeed, this point was illustrated during a news conference held by Defence General Counsel William Haynes on 21 March 2002. In response to questions about whether those detainees who were acquitted of crimes would be set free, Haynes remarked, 'The people that we now hold at Guantanamo are held for a specific reason that is not tied specifically to any particular crime. They're not held—they're not being held on the basis that they are necessarily criminals' (qtd. in Butler *Precarious Life* 75). In the narrative structure of the War on Terror that such a remark illuminates, it is clear that the term 'terrorist' and its synonyms references a politico-rhetorical reality rather than a strictly legal one, and moreover justifies a host of antagonistic and dehumanising strategies.

What matters particularly here are the consequences of this appellation for those so named who want to testify to torture (or speak as witnesses for others). In this context, not only do 'terrorists' occupy the shadowy border of the non-human, but they are also incapable of producing truthful speech about their injuries. This view supposedly derives from an Al Qaeda manual seized in a British raid on a cell in Manchester, in which operatives are encouraged to 'complain of mistreatment' should they be captured (The Washington Times). In a discursive slippage, it is then held that all such persons designated as 'terrorists', however spuriously, must be committed to exercising precisely this tactic. The Pentagon applied just such a strategy in its response to the *Washington Post* article that documented Mamdouh Habib's claims of torture. A spokesman reported that Habib's testimony 'fit the standard operating procedure' documented in Al Qaeda's training manuals (Mayer 9). On this model, the person who is designated as a terrorist is unable to produce credible speech about human rights violations. Shortly after this remark—and only a few days after the *Washington Post* published an article documenting his torture claims (Mayer 9)—Mamdouh Habib was suddenly released back to Australia. Even though he had been detained for more than three years without charge, and no suspicions against him had ever been established, the Australian government insisted on immediately interpellating him into the discourse of 'terrorist'. For example, in a joint media release produced by the Foreign Minister and the Attorney-General, it was stated that: 'The United States considers Mr Habib to be an enemy combatant who has been detained in accordance with the laws of war ... It remains the strong view of the United States that, based on information available to it, Mr Habib had prior knowledge of the terrorist attacks on or before 11 September 2001' (Downer and Ruddock). By focalising Habib through the criminalising narrative of the United States, this document seeks to jam the circuitry of the human rights paradigm described by Schaffer and Smith: 'Storytellers ... .are expected to take up the subject position of 'innocent' victims; they are expected to be able to occupy that position unambiguously' (161). By spuriously reiterating Habib's identity as an 'enemy combatant', this document works as a rhetorical defence against any future account of torture that he might go on to narrate. From this perspective, Habib is thus positioned as an 'unviable subject' (Butler *Excitable Speech* 136) in the field of public debate.

It is important to understand that torture complainants in the War on Terror face not only rhetorical but legal problems when attempting to establish their testimony—legal problems which themselves have consequences at the level of narrative. The Bush Administration has produced a substantial body of rules, definitions and internal memoranda relating to torture since the terrorist attacks of 9/11—the so-called 'torture papers' (Green and Dratel). Jeremy Waldron in particular has powerfully exposed the exceptional breaches of international legal norms and moral expectations that documents like the August 2002 Bybee memo display. However, legal analysis alone cannot exhaust the copious activity of this collection of materials. In particular, it is important to see these documents and legislative acts from not only a legal but rhetorical perspective; that is, to assess them from the perspective of their attack on detainees not only as *legal* subjects but as subjects of narration (Slaughter). The 'torture papers' can be read as having just such an end in mind.

For example, consider a relatively early memo produced by the then US Deputy Attorney-General John Yoo in January 2002. This document stated that 'the military's treatment of Al Qaeda members captured [in the War on Terror] is not limited by Article 3 of the Geneva Conventions' (43); that is, the Article which prohibits murder, cruel treatment and torture. When cast into positive propositional form, this memo (which deprives certain persons of the protections of human rights law) effectively then reserves the right to torture certain persons. This memo thus creates a category of person who can be tortured.

Strikingly, while the pattern of the early memos worked to construct a torturable person, yet other memos operated to deprive acts of torture themselves of their conventional signifying power. For example, the infamous August 2002 Bybee memo[8] dramatically narrowed the definition of torture to denote only those acts which produced pain equivalent to that accompanying 'serious physical injury such as organ failure, impairment of bodily function, or even death.' (172). Such a redefinition of the concept of torture prevents acts such as sexual humiliation, the use of dogs and even rape from appearing within its ambit. While this memo has been powerfully critiqued for the flaws in both its legal and moral reasoning, less remarked is its attack on detainees as speaking subjects. It ensures, for example, that a detainee who had suffered extremes of temperature or mock executions would be unable to narrate that injury under the sign of torture. Indeed, the memo's tendentious logic suggests that, the only subject authorised to narrate testimony about torture would be subject on the border of life and death—the exceptional subject who has suffered pain 'equivalent' to death but without being finally vanquished.

The torture laws' attack on narratability and the speaking subject as such is more recently exemplified in the Military Commissions Act of 2006. It contains an extraordinary provision. As Michael Otterman explains, the Act prohibits non-citizens from filing any claim relating to 'their detention, transfer, treatment or conditions of confinement' (186). When looked at squarely, it is clear that this prohibition (retrospective to 1997) deprives a whole category of person—the enemy combatant and its synonyms—of the right to testify to and litigate their injuries, such as those that might be occasioned by torture.

Taken together, these legal innovations both create a category of person who can be tortured, while removing the possibility that such persons could prosecute their attackers having suffered such a crime. As well as contributing to the figuration of torture testimony as an 'inexpressible' utterance (Rejali 580), this legal predicament produces a case of the *differend*, as described by Jean-Francois Lyotard: 'This is what a wrong would be: a damage accompanied by the loss of the means to prove the damage' (5). The legal and rhetorical attacks on torture complainants described so far document the way in which speech acts are able to work on other speech acts; the way in which testimony (and the ability to narrate) can itself become a target of power. In the Australian context, it is the extraordinary plea bargain of David Hicks which illustrates these strategies most starkly.

After nearly six years in Guantanamo Bay, David Hicks was charged with material support for a terrorist act and for terrorism, in a cloud of controversy. In a remarkable series of events, Hicks's captors informed him of the charges that they were laying against him the day after his legal team had flown out of

Guantanamo Bay, and allegedly also after he had been forcibly sedated (Debelle 'Hicks Given Sedative'). According to his defence lawyer Major Michael Mori, Hicks reported being semi-conscious as a result of the medication and was not able to understand what was happening to him. While US officials denied that they had sedated David Hicks, they nonetheless admitted that he had been given a 'GI cocktail' that included an anaesthetic (Debelle 'Hicks not Forcibly Sedated'). The charges themselves created a furore in Australia, where public debate for some time had been preoccupied with both prolonged detention of David Hicks and the processes of the discredited Military Commission that was set to try him. Despite mounting opposition from peak legal bodies around the country—which argued repeatedly that the Military Commission process, which permited hearsay evidence and evidence produced under coercion, was profoundly unjust—the Australian government persisted in giving the Military Commissions its full support, and had the dubious distinction of being the only nation outside of the United States to do so (Howard).

In a tumultuous day before the Military Commission, Hicks finally pleaded guilty to material support for terrorism, but not the more serious charge of material support for a terrorist act (Hicks 'Pre-Trial Agreement'). Two out of three of his own lawyers were dismissed from the courtroom just hours before he lodged his plea, for refusing to sign a document relating to conduct guidelines that, remarkably, had not yet been written (Coultan). His lawyers were effectively asked to put their signatures to a blank piece of paper. In this extraordinary morass of legal fantasy and rules of fake or future writing, Hicks 'pleaded' guilty, insofar as that plea is meaningful, given its literally fantastic conditions. In return for his guilty plea and the production of a carefully composed statement (which will be discussed below), Hicks was sentenced to seven years of which six years and three months was suspended. The nine months of the remaining custodial sentence were to be served at the Yatala prison in South Australia (Sales 228).

The components of the plea bargain that are relevant here are those that target Hicks's powers of narration. From this perspective, consider the following details. First, the plea required Hicks to agree to a twelve-month gag order. While he would be physically detained until 30 December 2007, he was not permitted to speak publicly about any of the circumstances of his capture or detention until March 2008. His testimony was thus formally designated 'unspeakable' for the duration of this period, and indeed he risked criminal sanctions should he break this rule. In this way, even though he had ostensibly finished his sentence by the end of 2007, he was juridically deprived of 'a place in the world' (Arendt 37) from which he could generate not only a public narrative of his experience but also the coils of civic action that might arise from it, such as an independent inquiry or Royal Commission into his case. Crucially, however, the plea bargain did not just require his public silence—it also required the performance of specific acts of 'speech', such as the following:

> In making this offer, I state that: (i) I have never been illegally treated by any person or persons while in the custody and control of the United States. This includes the period after my capture and transfer to US custody in Afghanistan in December 2001, through the entire period of my detention by the United States at Guantanamo Bay, Cuba. *I agree that this agreement puts to rest any claims of mistreatment by the United States.* [my italics]

The target of this whole arrangement is David Hicks as *a speaking subject*. While prohibiting him from speaking publicly for a year, the bargain simultaneously *forces* him to speak—forces this strange, juridical 'I' to say that 'I have never been illegally treated' (when the domain of 'legal treatment' we know is disturbingly broad—witness the recent failure of the new US Attorney-General to unambiguously state that 'water-boarding' is illegal).[9] The problem here then is not the speech of David Hicks *per se*—because the exonerating speech act is legitimate and in fact required of him—but rather the problem is the possibility of independent, *oppositional* speech from David Hicks, which in this context is speech that will undo, rewrite and re-present the story of who he is and what has been done to him. The strange requirements of this pre-trial agreement answer precisely this anxiety: *you must say that we did not hurt you*. Traced through this text is the fear that what David Hicks indeed will say, if given the chance, is that the Americans tortured him.

But the fact is that David Hicks *had already* said this in his two affidavits—one of which was operative before a UK court at the time of his plea—which is why the terms of this agreement are so disorienting.[10] Essentially, 'David Hicks is split between two moments of enunciation, two self-cancelling juridical 'I's'. In the first (embodied in the affidavits), he makes the statement 'I was tortured'. In the second (embodied in the pre-trial agreement), he makes the both awkward and euphemistic statement that 'I agree that this agreement puts to rest any claims of mistreatment'—a statement in which the word torture itself entirely disappears and indeed Hicks himself as the explicit subject of the claim. According to the rules of the plea bargain, it is only the second statement that has any force: it is these words that will 'put to rest' any prior (or simultaneous) claims. But there is no 'rest' in these words—what could such a phrase mean, except that those 'other' words will be made to finally lie quiet, refuse to signify, somehow stand outside the economy of iterability and recontextualisation which is the fate of every utterance (Derrida *Limited Inc*). This second statement is supposed to trump the stream of *other* words to the contrary, the dense network of co-texts that support Hicks's claims, such as similar testimony from other detainees (Shafiq, Asif and Rhuel), eye-witness evidence (*The World Today*) and human rights reports (Human Rights Watch; Human Rights First; United Nations Economic and Social Council). The plea bargain (with its juridical force) attempts to enforce precisely this impossibility: it installs itself, finally, as the truthful words on the matter, the words about torture that are true in the case of David Hicks.

The paradoxes inherent in this arrangement were illuminated when the then Prime Minister, Mr John Howard, was asked to comment in an interview on the pre-trial agreement on the night that it was made public:

> PM: David Hicks says he wasn't tortured. David Hicks has said he was not dealt with illegally.
>
> Interviewer: He also filed an affidavit for the British courts and said the opposite.
>
> PM: People might equally say that somebody who has admitted to training with Al-Qaeda would say anything (O'Brien).

The Prime Minister's words here unintentionally expose the regress at the heart of the structure: if Hicks would indeed 'say anything', then his plea bargain is as doubtful as his testimony. From this perspective, Mr Howard's adjudication here is a politico-moral one. On display is a taxonomy of speech acts with differential force: those which *accuse* the United States of torture are illegitimate (a terrorist would say anything), while those that *exonerate* it are granted authority (even when a terrorist says it). On this model, the phrase 'American torturer' can only be uttered by discredited persons and is excluded from the terms of reasonable debate as the Prime Minister's describes it. Despite the contradiction inherent in this normative arrangement as noted above, the Prime Minister ultimately succeeded in securing his interpretation: despite intense public concern over the detention of David Hicks, there has never yet been a public inquiry in Australia into his words about torture.

As Gillian Whitlock has argued, 'the instances where testimony fails to gather force and demand recognition require attention if we are to understand the dynamics of life narrative as an agent of consciousness-raising and social and cultural change' ('The Power of Testimony' 143). As I have tried to illustrate in this article, tracking the dialogised network of responses to narratives of human rights violations can reveal some of the ways that such testimony can be deprived of its signifying power. What is critical here is scrutiny of the forces of subjugation and non-acknowledgement that can plague the articulation of traumatic narratives in the War on Terror and over-determine the field of responses that seek to answer it. The predicament of Mamdouh Habib and David Hicks makes clear that what is required is exposure of what Derrida has described as 'the practices of recontextualisation' (*Limited Inc* 131) which repeatedly works to cast doubt on their words (and those of others like them), thus consigning them to the domain of the inexpressible. These textual and performative practices are thus materially implicated in the system of human rights violations that has become visible during the War on Terror. However, the incessant movement of iterability which re-cites this testimony in inhospitable contexts also generates the possibility that these testimonial materials will not be permanently vanquished. And indeed, the context around the testimony itself is rapidly changing: as I write these final lines, the report *Broken Laws: Broken Lives* has just been released by Physicians for Human Rights. As Major General Antonio Taguba writes in its preface: 'There is no longer any doubt as to whether the current administration has committed war crimes. The only question that remains to be answered is whether those who ordered the use of torture will be held to account'. Such acknowledgement—which has the potential to bring torture testimony into the light of collective consideration—means that the narratives of Mamdouh Habib and David Hicks may still be cited in contexts of civility that are yet to come; contexts that might foreground the principles of ethical inquiry and reparation, rather than the painful idioms of denial, dismissal and dehumanisation that have so far captured their words and kept them in shadow.

Notes

[1] For a detailed discussion of Mamdouh Habib's public testimony and the attempts made to silence him, see Philadelphoff-Puren 'Genre's Judgment'.

[2] Australia's international reputation on human rights has declined since the 1990s, principally because of its exceptionally punitive approach to refugees and asylum seekers, and its policy of mandatory detention. For an outstanding discussion on the ethical consequences of Australian migration law on the bodies of the refugees who are its target, see Pugiliese 'Subcutaneous Law'.

[3] As recommended by the NSW Council for Civil Liberties in Australia and Torture: Torture Shadow Report. Prepared for the United Committee Against Torture. July 2007.

[4] For example, see the 175 page statement of three of the five UK nationals released from Guantanamo Bay in 2004 (Rasul, Iqbal and Ahmed, 'Composite statement').

[5] The Military Commissions Act of 2006 has effectively legalized the use of these methods (Otterman 12).

[6] In a well-known interview, former Secretary of Defense, Donald Rumsfeld stated that 'I don't know if the—it is correct to say what you just said, that torture has taken place ... And therefore I'm not going to address the 'torture-word' (Online Newshour 'Iraqi Prisoner Abuse').

[7] In the British case, officials like Reginald Mauling reacted by insisting that 'It was necessary to take measures to fight terrorists, the murderous enemy. We must recognise them for what they are. They are criminals who wish to impose their own will by violence and terror.' (Conroy 230). Despite this powerful disparagement of the prisoners concerned, not one was ultimately charged with a crime.

[8] This memo was leaked midway through 2004 and was greeted with immediate international condemnation. As a result, it was rescinded with what is now known as the Haynes memo issued in its place in December 2004. However, as Waldron has noted, the new memo retains critical sections of the original (1704). Moreoever, there is evidence that the Bush Administration has never entirely repudiated the perspectives revealed in this document—at his confirmation hearings in February 2005, Alberto Gonzales remarked that 'I don't recall today whether I was in agreement with all of the analysis, but I don't have a disagreement with the conclusions then reached by the Department' (Senate Judiciary Committee Confirmation Hearing 2005). Shortly after this remark, Gonzales was appointed as Attorney-General of the United States.

[9] President George W. Bush said that questions to Judge Michael Mukasey about the legality of water-boarding were 'unfair' because 'he doesn't know whether we use that technique or not' (ABC News 'Mukasey').

[10] At the time of Hicks's plea, the second affidavit was lodged with the Special Administrative Appeals Tribunal in the UK as part of Hicks's attempt to apply for a British passport. This case was abandoned after Hicks's guilty plea before the Military Commissions. Personal communication from David McLeod (from Hicks's legal team) June 2007.

References

AAP. 'Ruddock Doubts Hicks's Torture Claims.' *AAP Bulletins* 10 Dec. 2004.

AAP. 'Sleep Deprivation not Torture: Ruddock.' *The Sydney Morning Herald* 1 Oct. 2006. p. 6.

ABC News. 'Mukasey Confirmed as New US Attorney-General.' 9 Nov. 2007. 11 Feb. 2008. <http://www.abc.net.au/news/stories/2007/11/09/2087098.htm>.

ABC Radio. 'Witness Claims David Hicks Abused by U.S. Military in Afghanistan.' *The World Today.* 20 May 2004. 16 June 2008. <http://www.abc.net.au/worldtoday/content/2004/S1112199htm>.

Allard, Tom. ''How I Suffered': Hicks's Grim Tale of Abuse in Bid for British Passport.' *The Age*. 2 Mar. 2007.

Appadurai, Arjun. *Modernity at Large: Cultural Dimensions of Globalization*. Minneapolis, MN: U of Minnesota P, 1996.

Arendt, Hannah. 'The Perplexities of the Rights of Man.' Ed. Peter Baehr. *The Portable Hannah Arendt*. London: Penguin Books, 2000.

Bennet, Jill. '*Tenebrae* after September 11: Art, Empathy, and the Global Politics of Belonging'. *World Memory: Personal Trajectories in Global Time*. Ed. Jill Bennet and Rosanne Kennedy. New York: Palgrave Macmillan, 2003.

Butler, Judith. *Excitable Speech: A Politics of the Performative*. New York and London: Routledge, 1997.

Butler, Judith. Precarious Life: The Powers of Mourning and Violence. New York and London: Verso, 2004.

Butler, Judith. 'Sexual Politics, Torture and Sexual Time.' *The British Journal of Sociology* 59.1 (2008) 1–23.

'Captives Told to Claim Torture.' *Washington Times*. 31 May 2005.

CBC News. 'Harper's Apology Means the World: Arar.' 26 Jan. 2007.

Conroy, John. *Unspeakable Acts, Ordinary People: The Dynamics of Torture*. London: Vision Paperbacks, 2001.

Coultan, Mark. 'A Glimpse of Five Years in Hell.' *The Age*. 28 Mar. 2007.

Debelle, Penelope. 'Hicks Given Sedative Before Told of Charges.' *The Age*. 19 Mar. 2007.

Debelle, Penelope. 'Hicks Not Forcibly Sedated: Military.' *The Age*. 21 Mar. 2007.

Denbeaux, Mark, and Joshua Denbeaux. Report on Guantanamo Detainees: A Profile of 517 Detainees Through Analysis of Department of Defense Data. 3 Aug. 2007. <http://law.shu.edu/aaatinal.pdf>.

Derrida, Jacques. *Limited Inc*. Evanston, IL: Northwestern UP, 1988.

Derrida, Jacques. *Of Grammatology.* Trans. Gayatri Chakravorty Spivak. Baltimore: Johns Hopkins UP, 1998.

Downer, Alexander, *Interview,* 2UE Radio. 14 Feb. 2005.

Downer, Alexander, and Philip Ruddock. 'Statement on Mamdouh Habib.' *Joint Media Release*. 11 Jan. 2005.

duBois, Page. *Torture and Truth*. New York: Routledge, 1991.

Felman, Shoshana and Dori Laub. *Testimony: Crises of Witnessing in Literature, Psychoanalysis and History.* New York and London: Routledge, 1992.

Foucault, Michel. *The Archaeology of Knowledge*. Trans. A.M. Sheridan. London: Routledge, 2002.

Forbes, Mark, and Penelope Debelle. 'Cuba Detainees Claim Mistreatment.' *The Age*. 25 May 2002.

Golden, Tim. 'Military Taking Tough Line with Detainees.' *New York Times*. 16 Dec. 2007.

Greenberg, Karen J. and Joshua L. Dratel. *The Torture Papers: The Road to Abu Ghraib*. New York: Cambridge UP, 2005.

Grimshaw, Tracey. 'Transcript of the Prime Minister The Hon John Howard MP. *Today Show*. 20 May 2004.

Haynes, William J. Memorandum for the Secretary of Defense. 'Counter-Resistance Techniques.' Ed. Karen Greenberg and Joshua L. Dratel. *The Torture Papers: The Road to Abu Ghraib*. New York: Cambridge UP, 2005.

Hersh, Seymour. 'Rush Transcript'. *Democracy Now*. 16 Aug. 2005. <http://www.demo-cracy now.org/static/hersh_trans.shtml>.

Hicks, David. 'Affidavit.' *The Torture Papers: The Road to Abu Ghraib*. Ed. Karen Greenberg and Joshua Dratel. New York: Cambridge UP, 2005: 1234–8.

'Hicks's Pre-Trial Agreement (Full Transcript)'. *United States V David Matthew Hicks*. 26 Mar. 2007. <http://www.theaustralian.news.com.au/story0,20876,21486066–17281, 00.html>. 18 July 2007.

Howard, John. Joint Press Conference with Secretary of Defense Donald Rumsfeld. Transcript. 18 July 2005.

Human Rights First. Leave No Marks: Enhanced Interrogation Techniques and the Risk of Criminality. Aug. 2007.

Human Rights Watch. *The Road to Abu Ghraib*. June 2004.

Lyotard, Jean-Francois. *The Differend: Phrases in Dispute*. Trans. George Van Den Abbeele. Minneapolis, MN: U of Minnesota P, 1988.

Mayer, Jane. 'Outsourcing Torture.' *The New Yorker*. 14 Feb. 2005.

McClymont, Kate. 'Habib Aims a Suit Right at the Top.' *The Age*. 17 Dec. 2005.

McCoy, Alfred W. 'Outcast of Camp Echo: The Punishment of David Hicks.' *The Monthly*. June 2006: 20–29.

Moeller, Susan D. 'A Moral Imagination: The Media's Response to the War on Terrorism.' *Reporting War: Journalism in Wartime*. Ed. Stuart Allan and Barbie Zelizer. Abingdon, MA: Routledge, 2004. 59–76.

Nagel, Thomas. 'Concealment and Exposure.' *Philosphy & Public Affairs* 21.1 (Winter 2008) 3–30.

New South Wales Council for Civil Liberties. Shadow Report Prepared for the United Nations Committee Against Torture on the Occasion of its Review of Australia's Third Periodic Report under the Convention Against Torture, and other Cruel, Inhuman or Degrading Treatment or Punishment.. 27 July 2007. 14 Mar. 2008. <http://www.nswccl.org.au/publications/cat_shadow.php>.

O'Brien, Kerry. 'Interview with the Prime Minister.' *The 7.30 Report*. ABC TV. 4 Apr. 2007. Accessed 10 Apr. 2007. <http://www.abc.net.au.7.30/content/2007/s1890384.htm>.

Office of the Press Secretary. 'President Discusses Creation of Military Commissions to Try Suspected Terrorists.' *White House News Release*. 6 Sep. 2006. 22 June 2008. <http://www.whitehouse.gov/news/releases/2006/09/print/20060906-3.html>.

Online Newshour. 'Iraqi Prisoner Abuse.' *PBS*. May 4, 2004. 2 June 2008. <http://www.pbs.org/newshour/bb/military/jan-june04/abuse1-05-04.html>.

Otterman, Micahel. American Torture: From the Cold War to Abu Ghraib and Beyond. Melbourne, Austral.: Melbourne UP, 2007.

Philadelphoff-Puren, Nina. 'Genre's Judgment: Discrediting Torture Testimony in the War on Terror.' *Law & Literature* 19.2 (2007) 229–46.

Physicians for Human Rights. *Broken Laws, Broken Lives: Medical Evidence of Torture by US Personnel and its Impact*. 18 June 2008. 21 June 2008. <http://brokenlives.info/>

Porras, Ileana M. 'On Terrorism: Reflections on Violence and the Outlaw.' *Utah Law Review* (1994) 119–47.

Pugiliese, Joseph. 'Subcutaneous Law: Embodying the *Migration Amendment Act 1992*.' *The Australian Feminist Law Journal* 21 December (2004) 23–34.

Rasul, Shafiq, Asif Iqbal, and Rhuhel Ahmed. 'Composite Statement: Detention in Afghanistan and Guantanamo Bay.' *Global Research*. 10 July 2006. <http://globalresearch.ca.articles/RAS408A.html>

Rejali, Darius. *Torture and Democracy*. Princeton and Oxford: Princeton UP, 2007.

Rose, David. *Guantanamo: America's War on Human Rights*. London: Faber & Faber, 2004.

Sales, Leigh. *Detainee 002: The Case of David Hicks*. Melbourne, Austral.: Melbourne UP.

Scarry, Elaine. The Body in Pain: The Making and Unmaking of the World. Oxford: Oxford UP, 1985.

Schaffer, Kay, and Sidonie Smith. *Human Rights and Narrated Lives: The Ethics of Recognition*. New York: Palgrave MacMillan, 2004.

Senate Judiciary Committee Confirmation Hearing. 'Transcript.' *The New York Times*. 6 Jan. 2005.

Slaughter, Joseph. 'A Question of Narration: The Voice in Human Rights Law.' *Human Rights Quarterly* 19.1 (1997) 406–30.

Stafford Smith, Clive. *Guantanamo Bay and the Secret Prisons*. London: Weidenfeld & Nicholson, 2007.

Stewart, Cameron. 'The Unmaking of a Terrorist.' *The Weekend Australian Magazine*. 10–11 Mar. 2007.

Thompson, A.C. and Trevor Paglen. *Torture Taxi: On the Trail of the CIA's Rendition Flights*. Prahran: Hardie Grant Books, 2006.

'Under Suspicion.' Transcript. *60 Minutes*. 13 Feb. 2005.

United Nations Economic and Social Council. *Situation of Detainees at Guantanamo Bay*. 15 Feb. 2006.

Whitlock, Gillian. 'In the Second Person: Narrative Transactions in Stolen Generations Testimony.' *Biography* 24.1 (Winter 2001) 197–214.

Whitlock, Gillian. 'The Power of Testimony.' *Law & Literature* 19.1 (2007) 139–52.

Yoo, John. 'Applications of Treaties and Laws to Al Qaeda and Taliban Detainees.' Ed. Karen Greenberg and Joshua Dratel. *The Torture Papers: The Road to Abu Ghraib*. New York, NY: Cambridge UP, 2005.

From Grief to Grievance: Ethics and Politics in the Testimony of Anti-War Mothers

Cynthia G. Franklin and Laura E. Lyons

Google 'Cindy Sheehan' + 'Iraq' and of the 1,340,000 results, an inordinate number are links to vituperative attacks on Sheehan, charging her with treason, ugliness, neglect of her dead son's graveside, and being a media whore and a hypocrite, among other accusations. While the bulk of the attacks on Sheehan come from ultra-right identified sites, particularly noteworthy for their vulgar misogyny and nationalist cant, the left, however loosely constructed, has not been particularly quick tc embrace or defend Sheehan, despite her having captured the media spotlight in the summer of 2005. The vociferous reaction to Cindy Sheehan points to the contested place that the families, and particularly the mothers, of United States military killed in US actions since 11 September 2001 occupy in American debates about the 'War on Terror.' These families' political positions on the war are not uniform. Nor are their individual beliefs and actions always consistent with those of their now-dead loved ones. Their grief, raw and emotionally powerful, can be enlisted to support the war or to bring about its end. As people who have paid a certain price in this war that most in the United States along with those in allied countries have not, their speech commands attention, and as the case of Sheehan demonstrates, not all of it is positive. In a country like the United States, where the George W. Bush administration would have its citizens understand that 'supporting the troops' requires unquestioning loyalty and unlimited funds 'to win the peace,' the speech of those like Sheehan who speak against the war often elicits explicit censure in the form of discrediting attacks. Alternatively, as is demonstrated by the case of the lesser known anti-war activist Celeste Zappala, who also lost a son, such protest can meet with tacit censorship. That is, it simply never appears in mainstream venues but rather remains at rallies, or is telecast on late-night cable access and on-line venues. As we discuss, in either case, whether censured or censored, these women's testimony serves as evidence of the importance of the politically and emotionally affective terrain of the family in post 9–11 anti-war activism.

After her son Casey Sheehan, a specialist in the United States Army, was killed in Iraq in April 2004, Cindy Sheehan became one of nine founding members of Gold Star Families for Peace. In August 2005, she attracted international attention when she set up Camp Casey just outside President George Bush's ranch in Crawford, Texas, pledging not to leave until the Commander-in-Chief met with her to answer her insistent question, 'For what noble cause did my son die?' Thousands from across the country joined her or set up camps in sites across the US. In the two years that followed, Sheehan's anti-war activism included travel to countries such as Australia, Cuba, England, Ireland, and Venezuela. She published a collection of her speeches, *Not One More Mother's Child* (2005) and a memoir, *Peace Mom: A Mother's Journey Through Heartache to Activism* (2006). Initially dubbed 'the Rosa Parks of the antiwar movement,' her speaking engagements have included appearances with US public intellectuals such as Noam Chomsky, the leftist historian Howard Zinn, as well as celebrities such as Susan Sarandon and Joan Baez. On 26 May and 28 May 2007, Sheehan issued statements ending her involvement with anti-war activism and withdrawing from the Democratic Party, though she returned to political life on July 3 of the same year.

Numerous websites and blogs track Sheehan's continued anti-war activities and her vocal criticisms of the Bush administration and the Democratic Party. The volume of commentary on Sheehan is excessive—and excessively personal and nasty. Googling Sheehan's name in combination with the words 'crazy' or 'insane' garners 280,000 and 122,000 sites respectively; treason brings forth 165,000 sites; 'ugly' begets 158,000 sites; 'fat' is a term in 137,000 sites; 'bitch' elicits 122,000; 'whore' garners 58,300; 'cunt,' 9,440; 'Hanoi Jane,' 9,020; 'douche bag' calls up 2,400.[1] A search will of course, bring up sites multiple times, and also will include sites on which commentators are defending Sheehan against her attackers. Some of these sites might put together these terms in ways that are not referencing Sheehan herself. Even allowing for these factors, however, the figures here testify to the depth and range of the rage against Sheehan, and the particularly gendered forms it takes.

All this attention clearly registers Sheehan's large public impact. At the same time, running more academic searches renders primarily journalistic sources, and very little sustained discussion of Sheehan's activism.[2] When we have spoken of working on Cindy Sheehan to our colleagues, we have met with eye rolls, incredulity, and occasionally outright ridicule (as in the ultimate academic putdown, 'I just think she's dumb'). So too, came the oft-repeated and unwarranted charge that her grief was unaccompanied by recognition of lives lost in Iraq.

Why, we wondered, such discomfort and need to disavow anti-war work that for several months had captured sustained international media attention that, sadly neither anti-war rallies with hundreds of thousands of people nor the hardest-hitting leftist analysis had received? Why, too, do invocations of Sheehan so often prompt the question: what about the Iraqi mothers? For us, these questions triggered yet other questions about the reception of testimony when the witness speaks as a mother, and one whose testimony emerges from the loss of her child.

In particular, the reaction to Sheehan made us consider the role of maternal grief in testimony, especially when testifying becomes a form of political activism. At times, anti-war activism has relied upon family members testifying to experiences of loss and trauma for which there is no juridical apparatus to appeal to for redress; nor are such witnesses constrained by rules of evidence or the presence of an interrogating interlocutor. For this reason, the affective power of the witness and her testimony in the broader public sphere rests largely on her ethos and the ethical engagement of her audience.

At the same time that we became interested in tracking Sheehan's role as 'Peace Mom,' we began thinking about the ideological work that mothers were playing in the 'War on Terror,' and wondering why this mother, in particular, was attracting so much attention in a way that other mothers also giving their lives to the anti-war movement were not. Another founding member of Gold Star Families for Peace, Celeste Zappala, for example, has, like Sheehan, also devoted herself full time to anti-war activism after her son, Sgt. Sherwood Baker, was killed in April 2004 while providing convoy security for the Iraq Survey Group whose mission was to uncover evidence of weapons of mass destruction. Zappala, like Sheehan, grounds her public addresses in Christian rhetoric, but to very different effect, and to an audience that is a fraction of Sheehan's in size.[3] If Zappala does not attract the media spotlight that Sheehan does, neither does she draw the vitriolic criticisms. In part, this might be attributed to the different rhetorical register in which she works: for example, in her speeches on YouTube, she is often magisterial and always insistent in foregrounding the ethical imperative of ending the war. Sheehan, by contrast, will often unleash her rage and disrespect for a regime that has 'murdered' her child and shown no remorse. Moreover, Sheehan's politics are at times uneven or lacking coherence: undergoing a 'hunger strike' that is a liquids-only diet, she will blog about the difficulties of finding a Jamba Juice store.[4] At the same time, what remains absolutely consistent is her grief over the loss of her son and her righteous anger over a war being waged on lies that line the pockets of corporations. Although it is always problematic when one person comes to stand in for a movement as diverse and complex in its positions as the anti-war movement, to dismiss Sheehan for having wide appeal is to engage in a moralistic but short-sighted politics. Just as the overemphasis on Sheehan to the near exclusion of Zappala by mainstream media pundits is questionable, so too the temptation on the left to choose activists such as Zappala over Sheehan bears questioning. Regardless of their differences, Sheehan and Zappala are both part of the broad-based anti-war movement and through those very differences as well as their points of connection, their examples speak to the politics and ethics of testifying from a position of grief.

In this paper, we will argue that, as the left dismisses Sheehan on political terms, it ignores important ethical questions about voice and public speech that she raises largely because her politics are not sufficiently 'pure'. And yet, it is Sheehan's lack of 'purity' that accounts for her broad appeal; it is her ability to mix rhetorical and political registers that makes her effective at reaching large numbers of people. Such wide draw is also precisely why the right finds it necessary to attack both her person and her politics as the many sites generated on Google searches indicate. Whereas someone such as Celeste Zappala appears to meet more fully an unarticulated standard of political coherence, it is no accident that she has less of a following. However, the ethical issues both Sheehan and Zappala raise are in fact the same, and to dismiss those because Sheehan's positions on the war are accompanied as well by, to use a shorthand, 'Jamba Juice politics,' is a failing on the part of the left that is at once ethical *and* political. As we consider the political purposes to which the complex and often powerful testimony chronicling loss of family members to the 'war on terror' is put, we argue that it is critical to examine the different invocations of the family in these expressions of grief. We argue that, it is crucial to do so in order to distinguish in ethical as well as political terms how the family is deployed, or sometimes dismissed in such testimony. By analysing testimony by Sheehan, Zappala, and family members featured in Ari Fleischer's 'Freedom's Watch' television ad campaign in support of the 2007 'surge' strategy in Iraq, we address the following questions: How do grief narratives allow for the recognition of other people's losses? When do expressions of grief over the loss of a family member make one complicit with a disregard for the lives of others? Is grief used to justify policies that view other human beings—both American soldiers and Iraqis—as so much collateral damage, and that render the presumed 'enemy' as inhuman? What does it mean to dismiss grief narratives as insincere or politically motivated? In addressing these questions, at the same time as we strenuously argue against the insidious uses to which the right puts testimony about family grief, we argue with equal vehemence that, to abdicate the power of the family to the right is not only an ethical but also a political mistake.

Testimony and activism conducted in the name of the family brings out the difficult tension between, on the one hand, the ideological traps of family rhetoric and, on the other hand, the affective power the family so often mobilises in American public life. Although Sheehan's testimony is often incisive and moving, at other times, its invocations of motherhood uncomfortably recall notions of women that feminists have spent decades resisting, because such ideas are sexist and essentialist and also because they underpin heteronormativity. In fact, Cindy Sheehan, as a grieving mother—a blond, blue-eyed, crucifix wearing one at that—represents the heteronormative subject *par excellence*. Put differently, she looks like Bush's America, which is perhaps why that administration and its band of pundits have needed to demonise her so thoroughly. So, too her conformity to these heteronormative ideals can help to explain the opposition she meets from much of the academic left, where the family has undergone rigorous and thorough going critique as a hegemonic instrument of a patriarchal and heterosexist state.

Feminist and queer theorists have been at the forefront of such criticism. Gayatri Gopinath, for example, looks to a body of feminist theory that analyses the conflation of 'woman,' 'home,' 'family,' and 'nation,' to understand how 'Women's bodies, then, become crucial to nationalist discourse in that they serve not only as the site of biological reproduction of national collectivities, but as the very embodiment of this nostalgically evoked communal past and tradition' (468). As defences of the family and pressures towards heteronormativity become increasingly coercive in the post 9/11 era—witness, for example, the prison scandal of Abu Ghraib being attributed to the breakdown in gender roles—critiques by Gopinath and others against nationalist demands that heterosexuality be a prerequisite of 'good citizenship' have become even more vehement. In 'Monster, Terrorist, Fag,' Jasbir Puar and Amit Rai remark upon 'some obvious factors that constitute the heteronormative character of American nationalism that have been exacerbated in the current political climate,' and single out 'the heterosexual family narratives of trauma and grief' (125).

At the same time, these theorists, along with others such as Sarah Ahmed, Lauren Berlant, Ann Cvetkovich, and Andrea Smith, demonstrate in their work the necessity of taking on the affective power that institutions such as the family put into play. Given the multiple forms of material and emotional violence, non-heteronormative subjects have experienced, these critics most often focus on documenting and analysing how this oppression works, on imagining and identifying queer spaces of resistance, and on understanding the social construction of emotions, and the important ideological roles that they play. Rarely do cultural critics recuperate hegemonic institutions, although this has been part of the work of Andrea Smith, who examines unexpected alliances among Native Americans and the Christian right.[5] Even those critics who take on hegemonic institutions typically stop short of recuperating the family, at least in its dominant, white, middle-class form. This justified wariness in regard to the family is not limited to the academic left; within the anti-war movement, it takes the form of a particular discomfort with the role of military families. In a recent article in *The Nation*, Rahul Mahajan, a steering committee member of United for Peace and Justice, and publisher of the blog *Empire Notes*, remarks, 'the surge in American nationalism has led us to grant military families too much credence.' Mahajan worries that the prominence of military families, even those speaking against the war, can nevertheless '[feed] into a critique of the war that [is] highly patriotic and jingoistic ....' (Houppert).

These critics have been absolutely correct in pointing to the pernicious uses to which the family has been put, particularly in the wake of 9/11, and their insights are indispensable. At the same time, given its ideological power, we dispense with the family at our peril: we simply cannot afford to cede the family to the right. Moreover, for ethical as well as political reasons, we believe that, it is worth grappling with testimony by Sheehan and other parents who have lost children in the war. This is not to suggest that, all narratives of grief are the same, but rather to consider both the ethics of mobilising grief on behalf of others, along with the responsibilities that an ethical engagement with the nexus of politics and grief requires. The stakes for such work are high: addressing the affectively powerful 'family' can crucially augment leftist analyses that situate the 'war on terror' in a global economy and that thus far have failed to intervene sufficiently into the imperialist march of US forces from Afghanistan to Iraq.

In part, the stakes surrounding Sheehan (and others who speak as mothers) are so high because, as the controversies surrounding her make evident, 'mothers' have assumed a place at the ideological forefront of the battle over the legitimacy of the US occupation of Iraq. Mothers, in general, and Cindy Sheehan, in particular, have occupied centre stage as the 'war on terror' has waged on. In Sally Fields' 2007 Emmy acceptance speech, the actress stated 'If mothers ruled the world, there would be no God damned wars in the first place'—a statement that led to her speech being censored by FOX (Marikar). In the days that followed, Fields was likened to Cindy Sheehan. Michele Malkin, for one, commented, 'This weekend, I met dozens of military mothers in Washington, DC, who fervently oppose the Sally Field/Cindy Sheehan model of maternal submission and immediate surrender'. Although Malkin's rhetoric departs from the norm insofar as she equates Sheehan's activism with inaction and cowardice rather than with maternal betrayal, what is characteristic is her need to attack Sheehan not just as an activist, but also as a mother.

Rather than use family values in the name of patriotism, Sheehan draws on maternal rhetoric and brings together, sometimes to mixed effect, Christian rhetoric and leftist analysis in order to oppose war as an imperialist venture. The appeals that she can make to a wide audience, then, are multiple: visually she emblematises conservative America; as the mother of a soldier, she relates to other military families from a broad cross-section, including people of color; as a

Christian, she taps into various religious communities, both mainstream and alternative; and through her increasingly anti-imperialist discourse, she can speak to the anti-war left. At times in her testimony, Sheehan articulates her position on the war simultaneously through several of these appeals: 'I think that the strategy of eternal, baseless war for corporate profit and greed is bad for all of our children, born and unborn' (*Not One More* 118). Within the same speech that recalls Christian, pro-life rhetoric, she also exclaims, 'What we as moms need to stop doing is giving our children to the military-industrial war complex to be used as human cluster bombs: to kill innocent civilians and to perhaps die enriching and feeding the gluttonous war machine' (119). For different reasons, these various registers all provoke the right. They cannot afford an opponent who can potentially appeal to the Christian liberal middle and to introduce to them a quasi-Marxist analysis. It becomes crucial, as a result, to take her down as a mother because, she grounds her activism in that role and uses it as the basis for emotional connection to her audiences.

Discrediting Sheehan as a mother allows her opponents not just to make a political point, but also to reassert regressive or retrospective ideals of motherhood. The excessive attacks on Sheehan as a mother speak to women's place on the political stage and the anxieties triggered by the presence of a woman, Hillary Rodham Clinton, as a viable presidential candidate in the 2008 election. The campaign against Sheehan also becomes a means to reestablish a mother as someone who stays at home and out of politics, which is the province of the father/state. Cindy Sheehan is brutally punished for stepping out of line—called a neglectful and therefore bad mother as well as a traitor to her country. Moreover, Sheehan is charged with betraying her son on the grounds that he chose to enlist. In the blog *Wake Up America*, for example, Susan Duclos, a mother who expresses her empathy for Sheehan's grief, nonetheless, states, 'What I cannot stomach is a parent that "uses" their child's death for a purpose that goes against what the child stood for. Goes against what the child fought for. Goes Against what the child died for. To me, that is a betrayal. Disrespect.' Sheehan's objection to her son's loss of life and to the war are cast as acts of disloyalty to him in a version of maternity that would have mothers not only passively support their children's every action and desire, but also leave unquestioned the consequences, even if that means the death of that child and others as well. Such accusations have exacted a tremendous personal toll on Sheehan; she discloses that, her activism was causing mounting stress-related medical bills and divisions within her family. In a 29 May 2007 resignation email, Sheehan writes, 'This system forcefully resists being helped and eats up the people who try to help it. I am getting out before it totally consumes me or anymore people that I love and the rest of my resources.'[6] At the same time, her almost immediate return to politics pays tribute to her conviction that, she can turn her grief for her son into action, and that she can make his death matter.

It is easy to understand the right's needs to demonise Sheehan. Less efficacious is the way that academics and the left have so often quickly dismissed her. And yet, someone like Sheehan—who represents a shift in political affiliations, if not from the right, certainly from the middle to the left—tells a story of dissent worth hearing, especially in an era when the dominant narrative in the US is the journey from Red Diaper baby to neo-conservative. Moreover, Sheehan's ability to marshall the family in support of a critique of nationalism is important even as, through it she challenges traditional constructions of the stay-at-home mother: 'We as mothers need to stop buying into the load of misogynist crap that our children need our constant presence in their lives so they can thrive and grow' (*Not One More* 119). Countering attacks that connect and criticise her politics and her parenting, Sheehan works to prise apart the presumed natural connection between being a good mother and being a patriot, a position promulgated by the repetition of images of mothers and wives graveside receiving folded flags, and then retreating from the public realm to resume their work (taking care of homes and children, or grieving unnoticed) in the private sphere. If Sheehan does not manage an end to the war or explicitly challenge heterosexual norms, her example nonetheless speaks to how activism that valorises the family can contribute to calls for a variety of structural changes at home and abroad. To dismiss this contribution ultimately colludes with the right and their dismissals of Sheehan.

Despite Cindy Sheehan's now iconic value to the right, and the shorthand way they can invoke her to dismiss the anti-war movement more generally, she is but one of many whose loss of a family member has prompted their activism in relation to the war. Another activist, working from her position as a mother who has lost her son to the current war, is Celeste Zappala, a member of Gold Star Families for Peace, Military Families Speak Out, a Christian Peace Witness for Iraq, and a participant at Camp Casey. Like Sheehan, Zappala tours the country, often speaking with her son Dante, though generally to smaller numbers than Sheehan, and her speeches circulate in alternative venues such as YouTube. Indeed, Zappala used YouTube to respond directly to the $15 million media campaign by Ari Fleischer and his Freedom's Watch. Fleischer's campaign featured sacrifices made by American soldiers and their family members in order to support Bush's surge strategy in Iraq. Zappala's short response, 'Bring Them Home, don't be fooled again' has been viewed over 25,000 times, which represents tens of thousands of more hits than her eloquent address (also available on YouTube) in March 2007 at the National Cathedral, marking the fourth anniversary of the US occupation of Iraq. While both Sheehan and Zappala foreground the losses of their sons to the war, the kinds of responses they elicit, as well as the volume, are indicative of the divergent ways they hold their audiences to political accountability and call them to ethical responsibility.

More than Sheehan, Zappala insistently moves from the significance of her own grief as a family member to the losses that others—and not just Americans—have incurred. Although she meets with disagreement, her detractors rarely, if ever resort to the viciousness and personal attacks that Sheehan draws for her political speeches. For example, in the extensive commentary Zappala's YouTube video 'Bring Them Home' elicited, the nastiest remark came from 'patsagainstrats,' who opines, 'It didn't take long for the far-left to mount a counter offensive to the new Freedom's Watch campaign. They'll have this poor woman running around at the Code Pink rallies in no time.' If not a personal attack, patsagainstrats' comment is certainly sexist. Even as he protests with condescension against the politicisation of maternal narratives of grief, his remarks demonstrate how these narratives receive intense scrutiny and have become enlisted in ideological—and decidedly patriarchal—warfare. Zappala powerfully resists patsagainstrats' patronising characterisation of her as naïve, as she also insists on the singularity of her loss *and* on the significance of the losses incurred by others when she responds: 'I really hope you do not think of my family's loss as a 'typical' anything. We are one of the 3,738 American families, the man we lost was unique, loved, brilliant and irreplaceable. We are not any one other than who we are, a family that misses Sherwood and wants the war to end.' Never invoking her son's death in isolation here, as in her other speeches, Zappala keeps to the forefront not only her own grief, but also asks us to feel the enormity of losses that have occurred. Zappala's ability to conjoin her loss to those of others distinguishes her from Sheehan, who evokes emotion primarily over the death of her own son and moves from that loss to protest the injustice of the war. Unlike Zappala, Sheehan represents her grief as individual and singular. Sheehan preserves this orientation in her speaking tours by calling upon local parents to speak in similar ways about the children that they have lost to this war.[7] Such family testimonies are *ad hoc* commemorations of individuals that are not necessarily meant to paint a collective picture of loss. Zappala, perhaps, draws less personalised attacks than Sheehan because, she herself foregrounds her loss as but one of many.

Zappala's speech as a Christian Peace Witness for Iraq at the National Cathedral is further evidence of the insistent way that she puts her loss as a mother alongside those of others, a position that emerges out of an ethics of witnessing, one that requires always keeping the other in mind. Hers is not an instinctive model of maternity but, an ethical as well as empathic one. In this address, as she speaks as a mother, she argues that, we cannot send children off to war to kill the children of others we do not know. She not only considers the lost lives of the Iraqi children and the plight of Iraqi parents—a neglect of which anti-war activists speaking as parents are frequently charged—but she also reflects upon the damages done to those who survive war. These include, she notes, over two million Iraqi refugees as well as 'the souls of soldiers.' Zappala's sense here of herself as a mother defies the kind of 'mother bear' role that women activists often draw on or have attributed to them; rather she holds her audience to a higher ethical responsibility, making them accountable not just for their own children's lives and well being but for everyone's. 'Each one of us,' Zappala states, is

> a witness to this war and to our own complicity in it. When were we silent when we should have spoken? Whose eyes would we not meet to face the truth? Now we are prostrate at this altar, begging Lord, help us.... Peace isn't the easy way out. Its creation is the most confounding, the hardest thing we can do. Help us. We lay

> our souls broken open before you and question how do we follow your command to love each other? Surely it cannot be by mindlessly sending the children of others off to kill the children of people we do not know.

Zappala asks each person to take responsibility in a way that is double-edged—just as we are all implicated in the war, so too we all can and must contribute to ending it. When she asks, 'Whose eyes would we not meet to face the truth?' her question pertains not only to those Americans who refuse to see their enemies as human, but also to those in the anti-war movement who would diminish the complex lives and deaths of US soldiers and their families. Her language explicitly calls for people to grapple with and act on their individual consciences. By contrast, Sheehan's analysis frequently works at the larger structural level—she looks at institutions and questions of empire. Pointing to the United States's structural complicity by invoking oil politics, she lays the blame for the war at the doors of the US government in tandem with corporations, letting everyday Americans off the hook. She doesn't ask individual citizens to wrestle with our consciences and responsibilities in the same way as Zappala. Imploring us to consider whose grief we cannot stand to see depicted, Zappala pointedly asks in her 'Christian Peace Witness for Iraq' speech: 'Who do we turn from?'

Zappala's religious belief that, we must be responsible to each other and will be held accountable not just for our own immediate actions, but what we have allowed to happen, is suggestive of a humanism that neither collapses nor reifies the difference between self and other, and that posits an ethical engagement between the two as a necessary condition for justice. This invocation of complicity resonates with Mark Sanders' formulation of complicity as 'convergence of act and responsibility' (11). According to Sanders, complicity is 'at one in the basic folded-togetherness of being, of human-being, of self and other. Such foldedness is the condition of possibility of all particular affiliations, loyalties, and commitments' (11). Sanders' theorisation of complicity, developed in the context of the social and political legacies of apartheid in South Africa, emphasises recognition of this basic folded-togetherness as the basis for responsibility. He takes as a productive condition of testimony the ability for both the witness and her interlocutors to hold in tension the need to account for a specific death with the necessity of that death standing in the place of unmarked others:

> Advocacy is a version of the essential human foldedness whereby one can assume the place of another.... The aporia, of course, is the fact that when one testifies on behalf of a father or a son or a daughter one chooses a specific other over another and, as feminist critics of the truth commission observed, over oneself as another. In the same way, the dead are never simply *the* dead...it is always a case of a *particular* dead one. There is always, necessarily, a contamination of *the* other with *an* other. Demanding decision, such contamination is basic to responsibility. (17)

Zappala's strength is precisely that, she manages at once to choose her son Sherwood and to move from him to humanise the nameless other dead. Through her testimony, she achieves what Sanders describes as a process of contamination, and haunts her listeners with the spectre of a vast and particularised sense of suffering and grief in the face of which we cannot throw up our hands, but for which we must take responsibility. In the way that she involves her audience with such profound questions of and struggles with conscience, she provides a corrective to the left and what its insistence on hard-line analysis so often leaves out.

In contrast to Sheehan then, Zappala's politics emerges primarily out of her personal ethos and her understanding that her Christian beliefs require her to be a pacifist, to take stands against war. Her words and actions ask her listeners to rise above their sense of self-interest, and hold them to a higher ethical ground. Although also a Christian, Sheehan's activism is less tied to an overall ethical vision. Her insistent question, 'For what noble cause did my son die?' is a call for political change. Her folksy demeanor and stories from her son's childhood invite her audience to identify with her ordinariness. Sheehan expertly occupies the political spotlight, a position she both courts and has been assigned by the media, and this is both her strength and her limitation. Despite Zappala's rhetorical power and tremendous ethos, Sheehan clearly has much greater visibility. What this points to is, just how important are the grounds on which activists speak in a culture in which personality predominates. The ways that these women testify as mothers who have lost children to war are different; however, it is not a matter of choosing Zappala's ethics over Sheehan's politics, or vice versa. What the two put forth collectively is a form of activism in which the ethical and the political cannot be segregated nor one subsumed into the other. As with the ethical and political, Sheehan's and Zappala's forms of activism are connected and interdependent.

Sheehan's and Zappala's rhetorics and positions contrast starkly with that of the lobbying group Freedom's Watch, founded by former Bush administration officials and members of the Republican Jewish Coalition and the conservative think tank the American Enterprise Institute. As Founding member and former Bush Press Secretary Ari Fleischer explains of its campaign, 'For those who believe in peace through strength, the cavalry is coming' (Allen). As this statement suggests, these professionally produced ads—which feature American flags, and shiny images of white houses, rolling green lawns, golden retrievers, and nuclear families—link war and its 'sacrifices' to a peace that can only be achieved through more aggression and violence. These advertisements explicitly and speciously link the war with 9/11. For example, in one, a widow, Laura Youngblood, claims 'I lost two family members to Al Qaeda—my uncle, a firefighter, on 9/11, and my husband, Travis, in Iraq. Congress did the right thing, voting to defeat terrorism in Iraq and Afghanistan.'[8] In another ad, mother Vicky Strong, in urging support for increased military presence in Iraq, states, 'The price is being paid; don't give up. We've already had one 9/11, we don't need another.' In another, which interestingly has been removed from the website, a mother speaks of her lost son as having been 'deployed to heaven.'[9] On the one hand, it is all too easy to point out that, these ads neglect the lives and deaths of Iraqis, a blinding omission that is obvious and ethically reprehensible. On the other hand, what Sheehan and Zappala help us to think about are the ways in which the grief of these family members is real, and should not be dismissed. Nor can we simply say that, this grief is being appropriated by Fleischer and 'Freedom's Watch', given how directly some of the family members express their conviction that their loved ones died in the name of fighting Al-Qaeda and terrorism. Although such linkages can and should meet with the harshest of criticism from the anti-war movement and the left, such criticism needs to be accompanied by an ethical grappling with the difficult connections between grief and politics.

In other words, while we are indicating that the use of family members' grief in the Freedom's Watch campaign is insidious, we also want to recognise that grief as real. Regardless of the political purposes to which it is put, family testimony chronicling loss is serious, complex, and often powerful. We are not, then, endorsing or equating or saying that we cannot or should not adjudicate among different uses or expressions of grief or invocations of the family. In fact, as we have been arguing, it is crucial to do so, in order to distinguish in *ethical* as well as *political* terms how the family is deployed, or sometimes dismissed.

Freedom's Watch mobilises a vicious, hyperbolic version of family as a national signifier, one that has violent consequences for both foreign and domestic policy. The reprehensible uses to which the right puts family and family grief, however, should not lead to dismissing, dispensing with, or abandoning this potent ideological field. Cindy Sheehan and Celeste Zappala each participate in different ethics of 'grief, that resonates with Judith Butler's contention that grief need not be privatising nor return us to a solitary situation [that] is, in [a] sense, depoliticizing' (22).

Rather, as Butler states and as the activism we have been discussing demonstrates, grief can furnish 'a sense of political community of a complex order, and it does this first of all by bringing to the fore the relational ties that have implications for theorising fundamental dependency and ethical responsibility' (22). Although family is not one of the relational ties that Butler discusses, the activism of Gold Star Families and other groups like them release political and psychic energy not in the service of perpetuating violence and suffering, but rather to apprehend 'a common, human vulnerability' (30). Testimony by those who have lost family to the war on terror, wherever they are located, demands a challenging ethical engagement, one not found in censuring attacks or acts of censorship. In firing high-minded pot shots at the work of activists like Cindy Sheehan or overlooking the example of Celeste Zappala, we squander the opportunity to leverage the affective, rhetorical, and political energy they are generating for a comprehensive critique of the US government's self-interested disregard for the vulnerable, precarious lives of human beings throughout the world.

Notes

[1] This search was conducted on 2 June 2008.

[2] For one of the few exceptions, see Abrams, 'Women and Antiwar Protest: Rearticulating Gender and Citizenship.'

[3] We only became aware of Celeste Zappala's work when we appeared with her on a panel. Zappala represented Gold Star Families for Peace during the session, 'Resisting War: Activism by Soldiers, Veterans, and Military Families' at the American Studies Association meeting in Philadelphia on 12 October 2007.

[4] See, for example, Cindy Sheehan, 'Troops Home Fast—Day 6,' (http://www.politicalaffairs.net/article/articleview/3794/1/198/). (Accessed 13 June 2008).

[5] See in particular Andrea Smith's *Native Americans and the Christian Right: The Gendered Politics of Unlikely Alliances*. At the same time, it is important to note that Smith also critiques the violence of hegemonic institutions. For example, as a founding member of The Boarding School Healing Project, she has worked with other activists to hold boarding schools accountable for a long history of sexual violence in Native American communities. See, for example, Smith's 'Soul Wound: The Legacy of Native American Schools,' (http://www.amnestyusa.org/amnestynow/soulwound.html). (Accessed 30 July 2008).

[6] See 'Anti-war Mom Cindy Sheehan Gives Up On Her Protest,' CNN, 29 May 2007, (http://www.cnn.com/2007/US/05/28/sheehan/index.html). (Accessed on 30 July 2008).

[7] It is difficult for grief not to begin to sound rehearsed when audiences already have familiarity with Sheehan's story of loss. Her appearances include by-now-known stories of Casey Sheehan. Calling upon local parents is one way that Sheehan effectively keeps the emotional charge these stories carry powerful.

[8] The Freedom's Watch video ads in support of George W. Bush's 'surge' strategy in Iraq can be viewed on the Freedom's Watch Website, (http://www.freedomswatch.org/MediaCenter/VideoAds/tabid/73/Default.aspx) (Accessed 1 August 2008).

[9] We last viewed this particular Freedom's Watch video ad on their website on 2 October 2007.

References

Abrams, Katherine. 'Women and Antiwar Protest: Rearticulating Gender and Citizenship.' *Boston University Law Review* (2007): 87.4, 849–80.

Ahmed, Sarah. *The Cultural Politics of Emotion*. New York and London: Routledge, 2004.

Allen, Mike. 'Pro-war group launches $15 million ad blitz'. 22 Aug. 2007. 1 Aug. 2008. <http://www.politico.com.news/stories/0807/5479.html>.

'Anti-war Mom Cindy Sheehan Gives Up On Her Protest,' CNN. 29 May 2007 <http://www.cnn.com/2007/US/05/28/sheehan/index.html>.

Berlant, Lauren. *Compassion: The Culture and Politics of an Emotion*. London and New York: Routledge, 2004.

Berlant, Lauren. *The Female Complaint: The Unfinished Business of Sentimentality in American Culture* Durham, NC: Duke UP, 2008.

Butler, Judith. *Precarious Life: The Powers of Mourning and Violence*. London and New York: Verso, 2004.

Cvetkovich, Ann. *An Archive of Feeling: Trauma, Sexuality, and Lesbian Public Cultures*. Durham, NC: Duke UP, 2003.

Duclos, Susan. 'A Mother's Betrayal: Casey and Cindy Sheehan.' *Wake Up America*, 19 Mar. 2007. <http://wwwwakeupamericans-spree.blogspot.com/2007/03/mothers-betrayal-casey-and-cindy.html>.

FreedomsWatch > Media Center > Video Ads. Freedom's Watch. 1 Aug. 2008. <http://www.freedomswatch.org/MediaCenter/VideoAds/tabid/73/Default.aspx>.

Gopinath, Gayatri. *Impossible Desires: Queer Diasporas and South Asian Public Cultures*. Durham, NC: Duke UP, 2005.

Gopinath, Gayatri.'Nostalgia, Desire, Diaspora: South Asian Sexualities in Motion.' *Positions* 5.2 (1997) 467–87.

Houppert, Karen. 'Cindy Sheehan: Mother of a Movement?' *The Nation*, 25 May 2006. <http://www.thenation.com/doc/20060612/houppert/print>.

Malkin, Michele. 'Silly Sally Field Doesn't Speak For Me.' *michelemalkin.com* 19 Sept. 2007. 1 Aug. 2008 <http://michellemalkin.com/2007/09/19/silly-sally-field-doesnt-speak-for-me/>.

Marikar, Sheila. 'On TV "Extreme Caution" vs. Free Speech.' *ABC News*, 18 Sept. 2007. 1 Aug. 2008 <http://abcnews.go.com/Entertainment/Story?id=3618536&page=1>.

Puar, Jasbir K. and Amit S. Rai. 'Monster, Terrorist, Fag: The War on Terrorism and the Production of Docile Patriots.' *Social Text* 20.3 (Fall 2002): 117–48.

Sanders, Mark. *Complicities: The Intellectual and Apartheid*. Durham, NC: Duke UP, 2002.

Sheehan, Cindy. *Not One More Mother's Child*. Kihei, Maui: Koa Books, 2005.

Sheehan, Cindy. *Peace Mom: A Mother's Journey Through Heartache to Activism*. New York: Atria, 2006.

Sheehan, Cindy. 'Troops Home Fast—Day 6.' *Political Affairs Magazine*. 10 July 2006. <http://www.politicalaffairs.net/article/articleview/3794/1/198/>.

Smith, Andrea. *Native Americans and the Christian Right: The Gendered Politics of Unlikely Alliances*. Durham: Duke UP, 2008.

Smith, Andrea.'Soul Wound: The Legacy of Native American Schools.' *Amnesty Magazine*. <http://www.amnestyusa.org/amnestynow/soulwound.html>.

Zappala, Celeste. 'Bring Them Home, don't be fooled again.' *YouTube*. 1 Aug. 2008 <http://www.youtube.com/watch?v=SSWzoGGmpqQ&feature=related>.

Zappala, Celeste. 'Christian Peace Witness For Iraq.' *YouTube*. 15 May 2007. 1 Aug. 2008 <http://www.youtube.com/watch?v=ELo6VBDdfJ8>.

Index

Abu Ghraib prison scandal 172, 173, 188
affect: and Indian Partition 58-9, 60, 65
Afghan Girl: National Geographic photograph 153-5
Afghanistan: asylum seekers' letters 151-65; Operation Enduring Freedom 153, 154, 158
Agger, I.: and Jensen, 100-1, 103, 105
Ahmed, S. 58, 59
Alexander, J. 110, 111, 112, 113, 116, 121, 122
Ali, B. 151, 155, 159
Amnesty International 76, 77
anthologies: role 61
anti-war mothers 6-7, 184-97; betrayal accusations 190; and family 188, 189; feminist and homosexual criticism 188; Gold Star Families for Peace 185, 186-7, 191, 195; and military families 189; responsibility debate 193
antiwar mothers: and complicity 193-4
Appadurai, A. 92-3
Arar, M. 169
Art of Fact (praCh) 17
Association of the Families of the Detained-Disappeared: Chile 100
asylum seekers: Nauru letters 151-65
Atkinson, J. 144-5
Auschwitz et Après (Delbo) 49
Austin, J. 160-1
Australia: asylum seekers' letters 151-65; Chamberlain murder case 109-26; Pacific Solution 6, 152, 154, 155, 162; reconciliation 118-19; Spare Rooms for Refugees project 152, 156; War on Terror and torture testimony 166-83
Australian Department for Immigration (DIMIA) 157, 158
Australian Stolen Generations 5-6, 119-20, 122, 129-50; apology 143; cultural trauma 119-20, 122; *Little Children Are Sacred* report 143-4; maternal trope 131-3, 136, 137, 138-9; Northern Territories Intervention 143-4
ayai: Cambodia 13
Aylwin, P. 93, 94

Bakhtin, M. 160
Bennett, J.: and Kennedy, R. 3
Beverley, J. 47, 48, 54
Bhalla, A. 59, 62-3, 64
Bhasin, K.: and Menon, R. 61, 65-6
Borders and Boundaries: Women in India's Partition (Menon and Bhasin) 65-6
Bourdieu, P. 39
Brennan, B. 162
Bringing Them Home report (1997): Australian Stolen Generations 129, 132, 133, 134, 143, 144
Brodzki, B. 132
Brough, M. 143
Brunner, L. 86-7, 88-9
Burnside, J. 151, 152, 154
Bush, G.W. 185
Butalia, U. 57-8, 62, 64
Butler, J. 153, 169, 170, 195
Bybee memo (August 2002) 175

Calma, T. 143
Cambodia 4, 9-25; ayai 13; Choeung Ek Memorial 18; memorialisation 18, 20; pin peat 12-13; Tuol Sleng Genocide Museum 18
Caruth, C. 105
Chamberlain, L. 6, 109-26
Chamberlain murder case 6, 109-26; apologies 121; and Australian identity 119-20; compassionate identification 115; counter narrative life writing 116-18; courageous agency 115; religion 115-16; Stolen Generations trauma 119-20, 122
Chauvel, C. 130
childhood memoirs 127-50
Chile: Association of the Families of the Detained-Disappeared 100; Jose Domingo Cañas prison 98-101, 105; Londres 38 disappearance centre 101-3, 104, 105; Loyola/Neptuno torture centre 103-6; Movement of the Revolutionary Left (MIR) 94; National Commission on Truth and Reconciliation 93; National Stadium 94-6; organised forgetting 97; reconciliation 92-3; Tejas Verdes 93; torture and detention centres 91-108; torture sessions 102-3; trauma sites 5, 91-108; Villa Grimaldi 96-8, 106
Choeung Ek Memorial: Cambodia 18
Cleary, J. 61

Clinton, H. 190
Coetzee, J.M. 166-7
Collins, F.: and Davis, T. 138
Communities Against Violence Network - Indigenous Women (CAVNET-IW) 5, 75-90; anonymity 80; death of Marisol Padilla 82; depressing nature 81, 86-7; foundation 80; members' praise 86-7; and narrative reception 82-5; posting philosophy/choices 85-6; practical support 80-1; resistance and truth-telling 78-81; traumatic remembrance 81-9; and visibility 81-2
compassionate identification: Chamberlain murder case 115
Connerton, P. 109
Conroy, J. 173
Coorey *et al*, P. 143, 144, 145
Council for Aboriginal Reconciliation: Australia 118
courageous agency: Chamberlain murder case 115
cultural carriers 111, 112, 114, 117, 122, 1116
cultural trauma: African-American slavery 111; compassionate identification 115; counter narrative life writing 116-18; and cultural carriers 111, 112, 114, 117, 122, 1116; debate 111; life writing as trauma witness 113-16; Lindy Chamberlain murder case 109-26; model 110-11, 112, 121; Stolen Generations 119-20, 122; Yale School 110, 111

da Vinci, L. 141
Dalama: Memoirs of an Invisible War (praCh) 10
Dalama: The End is Just the Beginnin' (praCh) 10
Dalama: The Last Chapter (praCh) 10-25
Dark Continents: Psychoanalysis and Colonialism (Khanna) 65, 69-70
Davis, T.: and Collins, F. 138
de Bonafine, H. 100
Death and the Maiden (Dorfman) 106
Deer, S. 76, 77, 79, 81, 85-6, 87, 88, 89
Delbo, C. 49, 50, 136
Derrida, J. 179
Des Pres, T. 49, 50
Didur, J. 61, 66
Dodson, M. 145
Dorfman, A. 106
Downer, A. 169-70, 173
Dubin, M. 80
Duclos, S. 190
Duran, B.: Duran, E.; and Yellow Horse Brave Heart, M. 77
Duran, E.: Duran, B.; and Yellow Horse Brave Heart, M. 77
Durham, K. 151, 154, 155, 157, 161; and Nauru art work 161-2

Eng, D.: and Kazanjian, D. 60-1, 71
Eyerman, R. 111

Family Frames: Photography: Narrative and Pestmemory (Hirsh) 64
Felman, S.: and Laub, D. 171
Fields, S. 189
Finding Ali (Brennan) 162
Fleischer, A. 187, 191, 194, 195
Fogiel, E. 128, 129, 141
Follow the Rabbit-Proof Fence (Pilkington) 6, 131, 133-9
Franklin, C.G.: and Lyons, L.E. 6-7, 184-97
Freedom's Watch: advertisement campaign 187, 191, 192, 194, 195
Freud, S. 60, 65
From Nowhere to Zero (Austin) 160-1

Geertz, C. 27
Genette, G. 137
Gilbert, M. 91
Gillmore, L. 1, 48
Glauser, B. 28
Gold Star Families for Peace 185, 186-7, 191, 195
Gopal, P. 60
Gopinath, G. 188
Gray, N. 85
Greece: reconciliation 104-5
Gregory, D. 152
Guantanamo Bay 167, 168, 169, 170, 174, 176-7
Guhathakurta, M. 66-7, 68
Gula, S.: *Afghan Girl* photograph 153-5

Habib, M. 6, 167-8, 169-70, 171-2, 173, 175, 179, 180
Haladay, J. 4, 75-90
Haynes, W. 174
Hersh, S. 174
Heryanto, A. 44
Hicks, D. 6, 167, 168, 169, 170, 171-2, 176, 177, 178, 180; plea bargain 168, 176-9
Him, C. 19
hip hop: and Cambodian-American youth culture 9-25
Hirsch, M. 132
Hirsh, M. 64
Hitchcock, A. 142
Holocaust 1, 3, 9, 49-50, 60, 91, 92, 93; and childhood memoirs 127-33, 139-42; maternal trope 131-3
Home to Mother (Pilkington) 137-8
Howard, J. 143-4, 145, 152, 162, 168, 179
Hughes-D'aeth, T. 133

Humphrey, M. 121
Hun Sen 19
Husserl, E. 27

I: Rogoberta Menchu - An Indian Woman in Guatemala (Menchu) 47, 48
I Just Want You to Understand (ɔraCh) 16, 17
Indian Partition 57-74; and affect 58-9, 60, 65; affective haunting 64-5; Bengali identity 64; collective trauma 63; illegitimate babies 71; melancholia 59; nationhood and women 69; and partition anthologies 58, 59, 61-71; postmemory 64; psychical loss 68; recovery of women 69-70; refugees 68
Indonesia 43-56; certificates of non-involvement 49; competing 1965 narratives 44-6; New Order 43, 44; political prisoners 45; sexual violence narratives 51-3; testimonial contexts and secrets 50-3; testimonial and political purpose 46-7; Truth and Reconciliation Commission 43, 45, 54

Jedda (Chauvel) 130
Jensen, S.: and Agger, I. 100-1, 103, 105
Joas, H. 111
Jose Domingo Cañas prison: memorial inscriptions 98-100

Kabir, A. 61
Kahane, C. 131-2
Kamboureli, S. 61, 66
Kansteiner, W. 111
Kany, C. 52
Kaplan, E.A. 3
Kaprallski, S. 104
Kaur, R. 67
Kazanjian, D.: and Eng, D. 60-1, 71
Kennedy, R. 6, 127-50; and Bennett, J. 3
Keo, B. 19
Khanna, R. 65, 68, 69-70
Khmer Rouge 4, 9, 10, 11, 12, 13, 14, 19
Killing Fields: generational impact 14; memorialisation 4, 9-25
Kluger, R. 142
Kofman, S. 6, 128-9, 130, 131, 139-42, 144, 145

LaCapra, D. 1, 60, 92, 104, 129-30
Landzelius, K. 76, 79
Laub, D. 128; and Felman, S. 171
Levi, N. 130
Leys, R. 1, 2, 111
life world: concept 27-8, 37, 39-40
Little Children Are Sacred report: Australia 143-4
Londres 38 disappearance centre: Chile 101-3, 104, 105
Loyola/Neptuno torture centre: Chile 103-6
Luig, U.: and Seebode, J. 29
Lyons, L.E.: and Franklin, C.G. 6-7, 184-97
Lyotard, J-F. 176

McCurry, S. 153-4
Madonna and Child with St. Anne (da Vinci) 141
Mahajan, R. 189
Major Crimes Act (MCA 1885) 76-7
Malkin, M. 189
Manto, S.H. 60
Mapmaking: Partition Stories from 2 Bengals (Sengupta) 59, 63-5
Mauss, M. 159
Mehdi, M. 156-7, 158, 161
melancholia: Indian Partition scholarship 59, 60-1, 65, 67-71
Menchu, R. 47, 48
Menon, R. 59-60, 65-71; and Bhasin, K. 61, 65-6
Mesure de Nos Jours (Delbo) 49
Military Commissions Act (2006) 176
Miller, N.K.: and Tougaw, J. 2, 3
Mitterand, F. 129
Montealegre, J. 92, 93, 95-6
mourning 60, 65
Mourning and Melancholia (Freud) 60, 65
Mukhopadhyay, S. 64
Mwanza 26, 30, 38

Nagel, T. 169
Nandy, A. 63, 64, 65
National Geographic 153-5
National Library of Australia (NLA) 112, 113, 116
National Stadium: Chile 94-6
Native North American women: Communities Against Violence Network - Indigenous Women (CAVNET-IW) 78-89; and legislation 76-7; mainstream news coverage 77-8, 88; and Native sovereignty erosion 77; non-native exploitation of land 77, 83-4; tribal land and lawlessness 76-7; and violence 75-90
Nauru letters: *Afghan Girl* National Geographic photograph 153-5; Australian asylum seekers 151-65; Australian Department for Immigration (DIMIA) files 158; correspondence 155-7; epistolarium 152; gift exchange 155, 159-60; Moh Mehdi correspondence 156-7, 158, 161; multiple writers/addressees 160; and refugee rejection 158; related artwork 161-2
Neville, A.O. 131, 134
Nikolic-Ristanovic, V. 51
No Woman's Land (Menon) 59-60, 65-71
Northern Territories Intervention: Australia 143-4

Oliphant v Suquamish Indian Tribe (1978) 76
Oliver, K. 2
Otterman, M. 176

Pacific Solution: Australia 6, 152, 154, 155, 162
Papon, M.: trial 128
Patel, K. 69-71
PATRIOT Act (2001) 18
Pearson, N. 143
Pedro Rojas Brigade: Chile 98
Philadelphoff-Puren, N. 6, 166-83
Pilger, J. 14
Pilkington, D. 6, 131, 133-9, 145
pin peat: Cambodia 12-13
Pinochet, Gen. A. 92, 93, 94, 95, 105
Pohlman, A. 4, 43-56
Pol Pot 4, 9; death 19
Poland: memorialisation 104
Pollock, D. 50, 51
postmemory: concept 64
Power: Territory and Rice (praCh) 14
praCh 4, 9-25
psychoanalysis 1, 3
Puar, J.K: and Rai, A.S. 188

Rabbit-Proof Fence (Noyce) 132, 133-8, 142
Rai, A.S.: and Puar, J.K. 188
Read, P.: and Wyndham, M. 5, 91-108
reconciliation 104-5; Australia 118-19; Chile 92-3; Greece 104-5; Poland 104
Rejali, D. 167, 172-3
Renan, E. 20
Rice-Sayre, L.P. 48
Richter, L.M. 28
Rigoberta Menchu and the Story of All Poor Gautemalans (Stoll) 47, 48
Robson, K. 49, 50
Rudd, K. 143, 162
Ruddock, P. 155, 172
Rue Ordener: Rue Labat (Kofman) 6, 128-9, 130, 131, 139-42
Ruffins, F. 104
Rumsfeld, D. 172
Russo, H. 129

S-21 (praCh) 16, 17
Saha, H. 68-9
Salughter, J. 171
Sanchez, T. 85
Sanders, M. 193-4
Santner, E. 61
Scarry, E. 167
Schaffer, K. 120; and Smith, S. 46, 61, 78, 80, 82, 169, 175
Schibotto, G. 29, 30
Schindler's List 133, 136
Schlund-Vials, C.J. 4, 9-25
Schreiner, O.: epistolarium 152
Schütz, A. 27
Seebode, J.: and Luig, U. 29
Sen, M. 68
Sengupta, D. 59, 63-5
September 11th attacks 3, 12, 14, 16
Seulieman, S. 128
Sheehan, C. 7, 187, 189, 192, 193, 195; attacks 184-6; betrayal accusations 190; discrediting strategies 190-1; nature of appeals 189-90; personal criticism 185-6
shell shock 1
Sierra, S. 100
Smelser, N. 111
Smith, A. 76, 78, 188-9
Smith, S.: and Schaffer, K. 46, 61, 78, 80, 82, 169, 175
Soft Weapons: Autobiogaphy in Transit (Whitlock) 152
Sommer, D. 47
Sontag, S. 153, 155
South Africa: Truth and Reconciliation Commissions 122
Staines, D. 6, 109-26
Stanley, L. 152, 153, 155, 159, 160, 162
Still Alive: A Holocaust Girlhood Remembered (Kluger) 142
Stolen Generations: Australia 119-20, 122, 129-50
Stoler, A.L. 46
Stoll, D. 47, 48
Stories about the Partition of India (Bhalla) 59, 62-3
Stories (praCh) 11-12, 14
street children: concept 28-9; drawings 29-37; Tanzania 26-42; and urban space 37-9
Strong, V. 194
Suharto 43, 44
Sydney Morning Herald 118, 143

Taguba, Maj. Gen. A. 179-80
Tanzanian street children 4, 26-42; coping strategies 26-7; difference 39; drawings 29-37; glue-sniffing 33, **36**, 38; injustice 29-30; life world concept 27-8, 37, 39-40; police 34-6, **37**, 38; prostitution 30; and street child concept 28-9; theft 31, 33, **34**, 39; and urban space 37-9; work 30-1
Tatz, C. 97
testimonio: definition 47; euphemism and vague terminology 52-3; Holocaust 49-50; multiple subjects and subjectivities 48-50; narrative contexts and secrets 50-3; and political purpose 46-7; sexual violence 51-3; third person narratives 51; and truth 54; women and post-Suharto Indonesia 4-5, 43-56
The Great Escape (praCh) 14, 15, 16

The Killing Fields (Joffé) 10, 14, 17
The Lady Vanishes (Hitchcock) 142
The Other Side of Silence (Butalia) 57-8
Thrift, N. 58-9
Through My Eyes (Chamberlain) 113
Tomsky, T. 4-5, 57-74
torture testimony: Bybee memo (August 2002) 175; clean torture 172; detainees' power of narration 175-8; discrediting strategies 173-4, 179; early US memos 176; Habib case 167-8, 169-70, 171-2, 173, 175, 179, 180; and hard news reporting genre 170-1; Hicks case 167, 168, 169, 170, 171-2, 176, 177, 178, 180; hostile witness 167, 171, 172; inexpressibility 167; and official comment 171; plausible deniability 172; second person witnessing 171; sleep deprivation 172; terrorist labels 173-5; torturable person concept 176; torture papers 175; and War on Terror 6, 166-83; water-boarding 178
Tougaw, J.: and Miller, N.K. 2, 3
Trauma: A Genealogy (Leys) 111
trauma sites: Chile 5, 91-108; and memorialisation 95
traumatic memory 109
Trinch, S.L. 52
Trouvier, P.: trial 128
TUES (praCh) 16-17
Tuol Sleng Genocide Museum: Cambodia 18

Ung, L. 19
United States of America (USA): slavery amnesia 103-4
Unnold, Y. 46

Valdés, H. 102-3
Van Boeschoten, R. 105
Villa Grimaldi: Chile 96-8, 106; Memory Room 97
vulnerable children: and disposable mothers 127-50

Waiting for the Barbarians (Coetzee) 166-7
Waldron, J. 175
War on Terror: and torture testimony 6, 166-83
Washington Post 175
Whitlock, G. 6, 46, 151-65, 179
Wiencke, M. 4, 26-42
Wieviorka, A. 128
Williams, P. 18
Wolff, S. 27
women: and Indian Partition 57-74; testimonio and post-Suharto Indonesia 43-56
Wyndham, M.: and Read, P. 5, 91-108

Yaeger, P. 2
Yale School: cultural trauma 110, 111
Ybanez, V. 86
Year Zero: The Silent Death of Cambodia 14
Yellow Horse Brave Heart, M.: Duran, B.; and Duran, E. 77
Yoo, J. 175
Youngblood, L. 194
Yudice, G. 48

Zappala, C. 7, 185, 186, 187, 191, 195; complicity invocation 193; detractors 191-2; National Cathedral speech 191, 192-3; nature of appeals 191-3; religious beliefs 193-4

www.ingramcontent.com/pod-product-compliance
Lightning Source LLC
LaVergne TN
LVHW080653011026
849160LV00014B/1406